Praise for

THE ANXIETY AND WORRY WORKBOOK

"Buy this gem of a book when you are ready to face your anxiety and take the necessary steps to overcome it. Drs. Clark and Beck are leaders in cognitive therapy, which has the highest anxiety treatment success rates in the world. Everyone who has ever felt anxious will recognize themselves in these pages and gain new understanding of what drives their anxiety. Even better, each chapter is packed with worksheets that can help lower anxiety within days and weeks. This is your chance to follow expert guidance with confidence as you take steps toward a calmer, happier future."
— CHRISTINE A. PADESKY, PHD, coauthor of *Mind Over Mood*

"From world-renowned cognitive therapists, this hands-on, practical, step-by-step workbook can help you free yourself from debilitating anxiety and worry. Use this book as a daily guide to understanding and changing your thinking. Drs. Clark and Beck offer a clear and empowering roadmap for building a better life."
— ROBERT L. LEAHY, PHD, author of *The Worry Cure*

"A great gift to anyone suffering from anxiety. This book is accessible, is written with warmth and wisdom, and includes the most up-to-date cognitive behavioral strategies. Enormously valuable, it is sure to inspire courage and hope."
— PAUL GILBERT, PHD, author of *The Compassionate Mind*

"A valuable and accessible resource for the millions of people around the world who suffer from anxiety, especially those who have panic attacks, fear social situations, or are tormented by constant worry."
— RICHARD G. HEIMBERG, PHD, Director, Adult Anxiety Clinic, Temple University

THE ANXIETY AND WORRY WORKBOOK

THE ANXIETY AND WORRY WORKBOOK

The Cognitive Behavioral Solution

DAVID A. CLARK, PHD
AARON T. BECK, MD

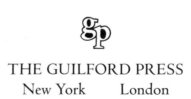

THE GUILFORD PRESS
New York   London

For Nancy
—D. A. C.

For Phyllis
—A. T. B.

© 2012 The Guilford Press
A Division of Guilford Publications, Inc.
370 Seventh Avenue, Suite 1200, New York, NY 10001
www.guilford.com

The information in this volume is not intended as a substitute for consultation with healthcare professionals. Each individual's health concerns should be evaluated by a qualified professional.

Printed in the United States of America

This book is printed on acid-free paper.

Last digit is print number: 9   8   7   6   5   4

Library of Congress Cataloging-in-Publication Data

Clark, David A., 1954–
      The anxiety and worry workbook : the cognitive behavioral solution / David A. Clark and Aaron T. Beck.
          p.   cm.
      Includes bibliographical references and index.
      ISBN 978-1-60623-918-6 (pbk. : alk. paper)
      1. Anxiety.   2. Anxiety—Prevention.   3. Worry.   4. Cognitive therapy.   I. Beck, Aaron
T. II. Title.
      BF575.A6C636 2012
      152.4′6—dc23
                                                                                            2011018515

All of the people described in this book are composites of patients we have treated for anxiety or are thoroughly disguised to protect their privacy.

Contents

Purchasers can download copies of the
reproducible tools from *www.guilford.com/clark6-forms*
for personal use or use with individual clients.

Preface

Anxiety disorders are among the most debilitating psychological conditions experienced today. Millions of people worldwide struggle valiantly every day to control worry, panic, fear, or dread. But often they find that the more they try to escape anxiety and its triggers, the worse it gets—and the narrower their lives become. Using this workbook can turn anxiety on its head and improve your quality of life. The methods in the following pages are based on *cognitive therapy* (cognitive behavior therapy), which has been shown in study after study to improve anxiety even when it has persisted (and grown) for years. In fact, this manual is the first self-help workbook for anxiety offered by the originator of cognitive therapy, Dr. Aaron T. Beck.

The power of cognitive therapy lies largely in its focus on the automatic, distressing thoughts that fuel anxiety. In this workbook you'll learn to recognize, evaluate, and correct thoughts that may keep you up at night but fail to alleviate your worry or solve real-life problems. You'll gain the ability to reduce, even prevent, panic attacks by identifying exaggerated or nonfactual thoughts about physical sensations. If you suffer from social anxiety, we'll show you how to test your preconceived notions about what other people think of you so that the interpersonal relationships that can make life worth living no longer seem threatening.

We wrote this book both as a self-help manual and as a companion to cognitive therapy guided by our treatment manual for therapists, *Cognitive Therapy of Anxiety Disorders: Science and Practice*. If you don't have access to a qualified therapist trained in cognitive therapy, this workbook can still offer hope and help. Work through the first eight chapters of the book, and if you feel you need more focused help with panic, social anxiety, or worry, continue to Chapters 9–11. At the back of the book you'll find a wealth of additional resources—books that offer more information and advice, and organizations that provide support and can help you locate a qualified therapist should you decide that self-help is not enough.

Anxiety has many faces, but the dedicated work of hundreds of mental health researchers and clinicians over the last three decades has greatly enhanced the scope and effectiveness of cognitive therapy in dealing with the complexity of this condition.

This book is informed by the work done by many colleagues over those years, but in its essence it represents the combined research and clinical experience of its authors—Aaron T. Beck, the founder of cognitive therapy, and David A. Clark, a professor and clinical psychologist with more than 25 years of research and clinical experience in cognitive therapy for anxiety and depression.

This book would not have been possible without the invaluable contributions and encouragement of the staff at The Guilford Press. We are especially grateful to Chris Benton, who critiqued earlier drafts of the manuscript and offered extensive revisions on every chapter. Her creativity, wisdom, efficiency, and enthusiasm as our developmental editor were critical to the completion of this project. It was truly a pleasure to work with Chris, who so freely shared with us her expertise in knowledge translation. We also appreciate the support, encouragement, and vision of our editor, Kitty Moore, who has been a strong advocate and provided valuable editorial assistance throughout the development of the workbook. Working closely on this project with Kitty and Chris has been a highly positive, enriching, and collaborative process that has led to a text far better than we could produce by ourselves. Finally, we wish to acknowledge the contribution of numerous colleagues who over the years have made an enormous contribution to the development of cognitive therapy, to our students who continue to enrich our knowledge, and to our patients who have taught us much about living with anxiety.

1

Making a New Start

We all know what it feels like to be afraid when confronted by a threatening stranger on the street, or to be anxious before an important exam or job interview, or to worry about the outcome of a medical test. It's hard to imagine living in a state of perpetual calm and safety, free from uncertainty, risk, danger, or threats. Fear and anxiety are part of living—and often a useful part, at that. Fear warns us of an impending danger, like when we feel the car slide on a wet or icy road or when a suspicious stranger appears to be following us. Feeling anxious can motivate a person to be better prepared for an important business meeting or take extra precautions when traveling to an unfamiliar place. The fact is, we need some fear and anxiety in our lives.

> Fear and anxiety are as normal as eating, sleeping, and breathing. Since we need them for survival, it would be dangerous to eliminate all fear and anxiety from life.

But not all fear and anxiety experiences are good for us. As a psychologist (D. A. C.) and a psychiatrist (A. T. B.), we've heard thousands of stories about individuals' daily struggles to contain their fears and anxiety. For some people anxiety becomes overwhelming, characterized by excessive and persistent feelings of apprehension, worry, tension, and nervousness over everyday situations that most people face with little concern.

Worried to Death

Rebecca can't sleep. In the past 5 years since being promoted to store manager, this 38-year-old mother of two school-age daughters has been fraught with apprehension, nervousness, and worries over her work, her children's safety, her aging parents' health, personal finances, and her husband's job insecurities. Her mind seems to generate an endless list of possible catastrophes—she won't be an effective manager at work, she'll fail to meet monthly sales projections, her younger daughter will get injured at school or her older daughter will be teased by friends, her parents will be disappointed in her for not visiting them, she won't have enough money left over after paying bills to contribute to their retirement savings plan, her husband could lose his job any day ... the list goes on. Rebecca has always been a worrier, but it has become almost unbearable in the last few years. In addition to sleepless nights, Rebecca finds that she is almost constantly agitated, shaky, "rattled," unable to relax, and irritable, with occasional anger outbursts. She breaks down in tears for no apparent reason. The worries are relentless and impossible to control. Despite her best efforts at distraction and reassuring herself that everything will be fine, she has a sick feeling in her stomach that "everything is going to come unraveled."

If you also tend to worry, note a few ways your experience is similar to or different from Rebecca's.

_____

_____

Losing His Grip

Todd is losing control—at least that's how it seems to him. As a recent college graduate starting a new job in sales, Todd had just moved to a new city and for the first time had his own apartment. He was making friends; he had a steady girlfriend, and he was making great progress in his new occupation. His initial performance evaluations were extremely positive. Life was good; but all this suddenly changed for Todd on a cool November day while driving home from work. His job had been somewhat stressful, with Todd working extra hours to finish a large client project on time. He had gone to the gym afterward to do his cardio routine and work off some of the stress of the day. On his way home a strange and unexpected feeling overtook Todd. Suddenly his chest tightened and his heart started pounding rapidly. He felt lightheaded, almost dizzy, as if he was about to faint. He pulled off to the side of the road, turned off the car, and gripped the wheel. By now he was feeling tense and started to shake and tremble. He felt extremely hot and started gasping for breath, convinced he was suffocating. Instantly, Todd wondered whether he was having a heart attack, just like his uncle had had 3 years earlier. He waited a few minutes until the symptoms settled down and then drove to the emergency room. A thorough examination and medical tests revealed no physical problems. The attending physician called it a panic attack, gave Todd an Ativan, and told him to see his family doctor.

That first attack happened 9 months ago, and since then Todd's life has changed dramatically. He now has frequent panic attacks and is almost constantly worried about his health. He has cut back on social activities and now finds he is afraid to go places for fear of having another attack. He restricts himself to work, his girlfriend's apartment, and his own place, afraid to venture into new or unfamiliar territory. Todd's world has shrunk, dominated by fear and avoidance.

If you've had panic attacks, how do they compare to Todd's experience?

_____

_____

Dying of Embarrassment

Elizabeth is a painfully shy single woman in her mid-40s. Since childhood she has always felt anxious around other people and so avoids social interaction as much as possible. It seems like just about everything to do with other people makes her anxious—carrying on a conversation, answering the phone, speaking up in a meeting, asking a store clerk for assistance, even eating in a restaurant or walking up the aisle of a movie theater. All of these situations make her feel tense, anxious, and self-conscious as she worries about blushing and coming across as awkward. She's convinced that people are always looking at her and wondering what's wrong with her. On occasions she has had panic attacks and has felt incredibly embarrassed by her behavior in social settings. As a result, Elizabeth avoids social and public situations as much as possible. She has only one close friend and spends most weekends with her aging parents. Although very competent in her job as an office clerk, she has been overlooked for promotion because of her awkwardness around others. Elizabeth is caught in her own little world, feeling depressed, lonely, and unloved—trapped by her fears and anxiety over people.

If you feel anxious around people, how does it compare with Elizabeth's experience?

_____

_____

Rebecca, Todd, and Elizabeth all experienced intense and persistent anxiety that caused significant distress and interference in their lives. Given that you've started reading this workbook, it is likely that fear and anxiety are causing a problem for you as well. Fortunately for the three individuals you just read about, each of them was able to make a new start by learning how to use proven psychological strategies to overcome debilitating anxiety. In this workbook we share with you numerous approaches that are used by effective therapists in their treatment of anxiety and its disorders. As will be evident, you too can begin afresh with greater understanding and more effective strategies that will enable you to overcome the burden of anxiety.

You're Not Alone

More than 65 million American adults will experience a clinically significant anxiety condition sometime in their life, making it *the most common mental health problem*.[1] In other words, more than one-quarter of your friends, colleagues, and neighbors will have some experience of severe anxiety, even if the majority don't seek professional help. Some well-known and successful people have struggled with anxiety, including Kim Basinger, Nicolas Cage, Winston Churchill, Abraham Lincoln, Howie Mandel, Donny Osmond, Barbra Streisand, and Howard Stern.[2] So there is no reason to be embarrassed or to blame yourself for your fears and anxiety. You certainly are not alone in your struggles. The good news is that in the last two decades mental health researchers have made great strides in advancing our knowledge and treatment of anxiety disorders. Help is available that can significantly reduce the intensity, persistence, and negative effects of your anxiety.

How Can This Workbook Help?

You can use this workbook on your own, but in our experience the methods you'll be using are even more effective when used in therapy with an experienced mental health professional. The methods in this book are based on *cognitive therapy* (CT), which was first developed in the 1960s by one of us (Aaron T. Beck) for the treatment of depression.[3] In 1985 Beck and his colleagues published *Anxiety Disorders and Phobias: A Cognitive Perspective,* which outlined a new version of *cognitive therapy* for the treatment of anxiety.[4] In 2010 we refined and updated the therapy in *Cognitive Therapy of Anxiety Disorders: Science and Practice* based on scientific findings on the nature and treatment of anxiety made in the last 25 years.[5]

Today *cognitive therapy* (or cognitive behavior therapy [CBT]) is practiced by hundreds of mental health practitioners worldwide and has been shown in dozens of scientific clinical outcome studies to be an effective treatment for many forms of anxiety disorder: 60–80% of people with an anxiety problem who complete a course of cognitive therapy (i.e., 10–20 sessions) will experience a significant reduction in their anxiety, although only a minority (i.e., 25–40%) will be completely symptom free.[6,7] This is equivalent to or better than the effectiveness of medication alone, but in a number of studies cognitive therapy produced longer-lasting improvement than medication alone.[8] Cognitive behavior

> Thousands of people with anxiety are living testimony that a person can live a productive and satisfying life even with significant periods of distress. You too *can* reduce the intensity, persistence, and negative effects of anxiety in your life. It is possible to "put the genie back in the bottle," to return fear and anxiety to their normal, rightful place in your life.

therapy is substantially more effective for anxiety than doing nothing or getting basic supportive counseling. Because of their known effectiveness, cognitive behavior therapies are now recommended as one of the first-choice treatments for anxiety by the American Psychiatric Association,[9] the American Psychological Association,[10] and the British National Health Service.[11]

What Is Cognitive Therapy?

The term *cognitive* refers to the act of knowing or recognizing our experiences. So cognitive therapy is an organized, systematic psychological treatment that teaches people how to change the thoughts, beliefs, and attitudes that play an important role in negative emotional states like anxiety or depression. The basic idea in cognitive therapy is that *the way we think influences the way we feel, and therefore changing how we think can change how we feel.* The basic idea of the therapy can be expressed in the following way:

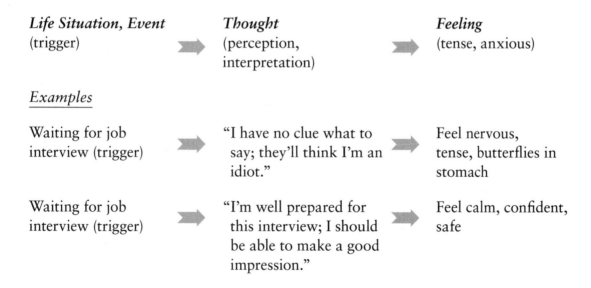

Life Situation, Event (trigger)	→	**Thought** (perception, interpretation)	→	**Feeling** (tense, anxious)

Examples

Waiting for job interview (trigger)	→	"I have no clue what to say; they'll think I'm an idiot."	→	Feel nervous, tense, butterflies in stomach
Waiting for job interview (trigger)	→	"I'm well prepared for this interview; I should be able to make a good impression."	→	Feel calm, confident, safe

Cognitive therapy is a brief, highly structured talk therapy that focuses on everyday experiences to teach individuals how to change their emotional thinking and beliefs through systematic evaluation and behavioral action plans— with the aim of reducing distressing conditions like anxiety and depression.

It's likely that you're thinking about your fear and anxiety as you read this book. To start practicing the cognitive therapy focus on "how we think," see if you can capture **what you're feeling and thinking at this very moment.**

At this moment I am feeling _____

At this moment I am thinking _____

_____

What to Expect from a Cognitive Therapist

If you have severe anxiety and you've struggled with it for many years, you may find it necessary to seek out a qualified cognitive therapist to get maximum benefit from the cognitive therapy approach. You can use this workbook as a companion volume while your therapist uses our professional text *Cognitive Therapy of Anxiety Disorders,*[5] which explains to therapists how to conduct cognitive therapy sessions for anxiety disorders. (As mentioned earlier, the workbook has been written so you can also use it on your own.) Even if you're not already working with a therapist, you might want to know more about what cognitive therapy is like.

A course of therapy for an anxiety disorder ranges from 6 to 20 individual sessions normally offered weekly at the beginning and then tapering to biweekly and then monthly sessions. There are three phases to treatment:

■ **Assessment.** The first session or two focuses on assessing the nature of your anxiety problem. The therapist will ask lots of questions about the history of your anxiety, its symptoms, your everyday experiences with it, and how you've tried to cope. Most cognitive therapists also give clients questionnaires to complete at home. The goal of the assessment is to understand the nature of your anxiety and develop a treatment plan that will work for you.

■ **Intervention.** This is the main part of cognitive therapy, which focuses on identifying the problematic thinking that is making you anxious, correcting these thoughts, helping you discover a new perspective on anxiety, and structuring action plans that will alter how you deal with episodes of anxiety.

■ **Termination.** The final few sessions occur less frequently and focus on skills necessary for dealing with the occasional return of anxiety. Therapists refer to this as relapse prevention, and its goal is to ensure the person has the ability to cope with future experiences of anxiety without therapist assistance.

TABLE 1.1. **Structure of a Typical Cognitive Therapy Session**

Session item	Description
1. Weekly review and anxiety check	Each session begins with the client providing a brief report on any anxiety-relevant experiences during the week as well as a rating of the frequency and intensity of anxiety episodes. (5–10 minutes)
2. Set session agenda	The therapist and client together set an agenda of issues for the therapy session. (5 minutes)
3. Evaluate previous session action plan	The results or outcome of the last session action plan are discussed and evaluated. What has the client learned from doing this between-sessions task? How can this be incorporated into a strategy for reducing anxiety? (10 minutes)
4. Primary session topic(s)	The main part of the session focuses on identifying, evaluating, and modifying specific problematic thoughts, beliefs, and behaviors that maintain anxiety. (20 minutes)
5. Develop action plan	An action plan is developed that the client does as homework between sessions. The action plan is based on the outcome of the "primary session topic." (10 minutes)
6. Session summary and feedback	The client provides a summary of the main points of the session and feedback on what she found most and least helpful. (5 minutes)

Cognitive therapy sessions follow a fairly typical structure, which is explained in Table 1.1.[12] Although cognitive therapists differ on how strictly they adhere to this session format, most elements, if not all, will be present during most therapy sessions for anxiety.

In addition, cognitive behavior therapists adopt a particular therapeutic style that they believe provides the best context for learning how to overcome anxiety. These characteristics are summarized in Table 1.2.[13] This therapeutic style, along with the characteristics of a good therapeutic relationship (trust, confidence in therapist's understanding, demonstrated concern and empathy, ease of self-disclosure, assurance of confidentiality), produces the best therapeutic environment for treatment of fear and anxiety.

Many mental health professionals have adopted elements of cognitive therapy into their practices, but only a few practitioners routinely offer a complete course of cognitive therapy or are formally trained as cognitive therapists. So how can you know whether your therapist is a cognitive therapist? The easiest way is to determine whether your therapist has formal certification in cognitive therapy through the

TABLE 1.2. Therapeutic Style Adopted by Cognitive Therapists

Characteristic	Explanation
• Education	Learning is a fundamental feature of cognitive therapy. The therapist assumes the role of consultant or teacher, who provides guidance and instruction on how to learn to overcome anxiety.
• Collaboration	The client is an active participant in the therapy process. Together the therapist and client set the goals and direction for therapy and work together to discover the best cognitive and behavioral strategies for reducing anxiety.
• Socratic questioning	The cognitive therapist poses a series of questions and then summarizes clients' answers to emphasize how certain thoughts, beliefs, perceptions, and behaviors are responsible for anxiety and its relief. ("What did you think was the worst possible outcome in that situation?" "How likely was this to happen?" "What were the chances you could have coped successfully with this situation?")
• Guided discovery	The cognitive therapist relies on probing questions to help individuals discover for themselves the root causes of their anxiety and how best to overcome it. The therapist avoids directly telling clients what is wrong or what to do but instead uses systematic questioning to guide individuals toward their own "cognitive self-discovery."
• Collaborative empiricism	Together the client and therapist develop action plans or behavioral assignments that determine the best strategies to reduce fear and anxiety. It is well known that change comes best through experience.

Academy of Cognitive Therapy (ACT). Currently ACT has more than 600 members worldwide—psychologists, social workers, psychiatrists, and other mental health professionals who have passed strict competency standards in cognitive therapy. You can find a certified cognitive therapist in your region by going to the ACT website (*www. academyofct.org*). A therapist without ACT certification may offer many elements of cognitive therapy or cognitive behavior therapy. Knowing what cognitive therapy consists of will help you decide whether a therapist you're considering working with can offer enough of the elements of cognitive therapy to help you.

How to Benefit from This Workbook

We wrote this book for people who have varying levels of fear and anxiety and to help alleviate, specifically, panic attacks, social anxiety, and generalized anxiety and worry, the three types of anxiety exhibited by Rebecca, Todd, and Elizabeth. If you identified with symptoms of any one or all of these people, you'll find help in this book. If you're using it along with a therapist, the therapist could use the workbook as a companion to your treatment by assigning certain chapters, special sections, or particular exercises that would enhance the therapy experience and help you make quicker and more effective progress in reducing anxiety. Many of the exercise forms, diaries, and rating scales in this book are modified reproductions from the therapist manual *Cognitive Therapy of Anxiety Disorders*.[5]

Again, you can work through the book on your own, although you'll get more out of it if you seek professional treatment, because working on difficult emotions like anxiety is a matter of not only knowing what to do but also learning how to apply this knowledge to your everyday experiences of anxiety. Either way, you'll gain the greatest benefit if you:

- **Have a significant problem** (anxiety is an important issue for you because it's causing substantial distress and interference in your life).

- **Are highly motivated** (ready to devote time and effort to getting better).

- **Have positive expectations** (expect you can make improvements in anxiety whether you're working with a therapist or using this workbook on your own).

What If You're Taking Medication or Are Engaged in Other Psychotherapy?

Many people with an anxiety disorder start taking medication (antidepressants or tranquilizers) before they begin psychotherapy. Even if your medication has been effective in reducing anxiety, you may want a course of cognitive therapy if you are concerned about a return of anxiety once you stop taking medication. In that case, your therapist and physician should consult with each other to determine the best combination of therapy and medication, because cognitive therapy is designed to help you learn to tolerate anxiety, not to avoid it, and many medications either eliminate all anxiety or are used specifically to avoid anxious feelings (medications like Ativan and Xanax are taken when you start to feel or anticipate feeling anxious).

If you are engaged in another form of psychotherapy, and it primarily concerns some other problem (such as family or relationship difficulties), you should have no problem simultaneously undergoing cognitive therapy for anxiety. But it's not a good idea to be engaged in two different therapies for anxiety, because the effectiveness of each is likely to be reduced significantly.

In our experience it's best to commit exclusively to cognitive therapy for anxiety over a 3- to 6-month period, either with or without medication.

■ **Can approach your anxiety as a learner** (willing to discover new ways to understand and respond to your anxiety experiences).

■ **Are willing to work on the role you may play in making anxiety worse** (it will be difficult to benefit from the cognitive therapy approach if you believe other people or your circumstances are to blame for your anxiety).

■ **Can be aware of and write about your thoughts and feelings** (can "catch" your thoughts and feelings and talk about them to a therapist or write them down in this workbook).

■ **Can take a critical, investigative approach to your thoughts and behavior** (are ready to use this workbook to look critically at the various elements of your anxiety experiences).

■ **Are willing to invest time and effort in completing action-based exercises** (i.e., homework).

You may be wondering whether the cognitive therapy approach can work for you because you don't fully meet all these criteria. We're not suggesting that you should avoid treatment or set aside this book if you don't feel like you measure up to these criteria. Rather these criteria are "readiness for change" indicators. People with many of these characteristics will probably get a lot more out of this workbook than people with only a few characteristics. A therapist can help you maximize your desire and ability to loosen anxiety's grip on your life, and this book will help you stay motivated and on track with various reminders, summaries, and troubleshooting tips (such as the shaded boxes you've already seen in this chapter). You may also find as you get into the workbook and do the exercises that your "readiness for change" gets stronger and your openness to the cognitive approach improves.

The best way to work through this book is mostly in order, reading the first eight chapters and then turning to the specialized cognitive therapy chapters that provide specific interventions for panic attacks, social anxiety, and worry (Chapters 9–11) if you need more help. The first two chapters contain a brief introduction to cognitive therapy and an invitation to take another look at your own anxiety. In Chapter 3 you'll read about the anxious mind—the cognitive view of anxiety. Then, in Chapter 4, you will learn about how cognitive therapy works and what types of exercises you'll be doing to address your anxiety using this book. In Chapter 5 you'll create your own anxiety profile, which will be packed with information that you'll use throughout the book's exercises so that you really target your unique problems and identify your strengths. **You should complete the exercises and worksheets as you read through Chapters 1–5 of the workbook.**

In Chapters 6 and 7 you'll learn the techniques that will help you lessen anxiety and its hold on you. We suggest you read those two chapters *without doing the exer-*

cises and then follow the instructions in Chapter 8 for putting together the cognitive and behavioral techniques into an Anxiety Work Plan that you can use to systematically carry out your cognitive therapy program. *Then* start implementing the work plan by doing the exercises and worksheets you've selected from Chapters 6 and 7.

As you read through the workbook, take your time. Try to apply what you read to your experience of anxiety. You will find plenty of exercises throughout and will get the most from the workbook if you complete the exercises. Above all, try to apply the strategies we recommend in your everyday life. Don't get too hung up on trying to do all the exercises and worksheets perfectly. You'll find some more relevant or helpful than others, and so you should spend more time on the exercises and worksheets you find most helpful. After all, the workbook is meant to be a practical guide, not an educational text. It is meant to help you "put the genie back in the bottle"; that is, to normalize fear and anxiety by returning them to their rightful place in your life.

Goals and Expectations

Take a quick look back at the "readiness for change" list above. You'll notice that we've already asked you to test yourself on recognizing and writing down your thoughts and feelings on page 6. If you had a hard time writing down your thoughts and feelings, don't worry! You'll get help with this skill and others throughout this book. Another theme in the readiness list concerns your goals and expectations. You'll get a lot more out of this workbook (and work with a therapist) if you can stay focused on your goals for minimizing anxiety's interference in your life.

So, before you read further, stop and ask yourself how you would like to change. Maybe you have been dominated by fear and anxiety, and all you can see is how it is wrecking your life. Well, what type of person would you like to be? What would you like to do that you can't do now? How would you like to handle fear and anxiety? How would you like to reclaim your life? What would you be like without excessive fear and anxiety? An example of a goal for behavioral change might be to speak up and give your opinion more often at office meetings, a cognitive goal might be to stop assuming that every time your chest feels tight it could be a heart attack, and an emotional goal might be to feel less tense and agitated whenever you think about retirement. Take a moment now to fill out Worksheet 1.1. Then come back to this worksheet once you've worked your way through Chapters 1–8 to determine how much progress you've made toward meeting your goals. If you're in therapy, you may want to discuss those goals with your therapist and include them in your individualized cognitive therapy treatment plan. **If you decide, upon reviewing Worksheet 1.1, that you haven't made all the improvements you want from working through Chapters 1–8, turn to any of Chapters 9–11 to do additional work specifically on panic, social anxiety, or worry.**

My Goals and Expectations for Overcoming Fear and Anxiety

Behavioral Change	Cognitive Change	Emotional Change
What behaviors would you like to increase? What behaviors would you like to reduce or eliminate? How would you act differently without fear or anxiety?	What thoughts and beliefs would you like to increase? What thoughts and beliefs would you like to reduce or eliminate? How would you think differently without fear or anxiety?	What feelings or emotions would you like to increase? What feelings would you like to reduce or eliminate? How would you feel differently without fear or anxiety?
1.	1.	1.
2.	2.	2.
3.	3.	3.
4.	4.	4.
5.	5.	5.

CHAPTER SUMMARY

- Fear and anxiety are normal emotions that are necessary to our survival.

- These emotions become problematic when they are excessive, persistent, and unrealistic reactions to normal, everyday situations.

- Anxiety is the most common mental health problem in America.

- New research into the nature of anxiety and its treatment offers new hope for those suffering from clinically significant anxiety conditions.

- Cognitive therapy is a scientifically supported treatment for fear and anxiety that is effective for 60–80% of people with anxiety disorders who complete treatment.

- The basic assumption in cognitive therapy is that we can reduce negative feelings like anxiety by changing our emotion-related thoughts, beliefs, and attitudes.

- Cognitive therapy is a brief, structured, verbally based intervention that uses logical reasoning and behavioral assignments to change unwanted negative thoughts and feelings.

- The therapist style adopted in cognitive therapy involves therapist–client collaboration, guided discovery of problematic thoughts by systematic questioning, and behavioral assignments.

- Individuals who have a significant anxiety problem, are motivated, and can become engaged in the therapeutic relationship will get the most out of a course of cognitive therapy.

- This workbook can be used to supplement cognitive therapy or on its own as a self-help guide.

Whether you're using this book with a therapist or on your own, the more you come to know about your particular experience with anxiety, the better you can aim your efforts at improvement. Let's start with Chapter 2, which will explain more about the nature of anxiety, what's normal, and what's not.

2

Understanding Anxiety

As stated in Chapter 1, everyone experiences fear and anxiety, and there's little doubt that some experiences would provoke fear in just about everyone. Wouldn't we all feel fear upon noticing smoke curling under the basement door, losing control of the car on an icy highway, seeing a tornado heading toward us, being attacked by an armed thief, or hearing a pilot announce that the landing gear won't engage and so they are preparing for a crash landing? Fear is a universal emotion that signals we are in imminent danger. As such, it's very useful.

But when fear is misplaced, excessive, and disconnected from reality, it no longer provides an accurate and reliable signal of danger. For example, if you had an excessive fear of dogs (i.e., a "dog phobia"), you might take extreme measures to avoid all encounters with dogs, even though most dogs don't put anyone in imminent danger just by being dogs. These specific fears or phobias can interfere greatly with the way those affected by them conduct their lives. However, fear is a basic emotion that also plays an important role in the more complex anxiety conditions discussed in this workbook.

What Is the Difference between Fear and Anxiety?

So far we have been using the terms *fear* and *anxiety* as if they mean the same thing. Cognitive therapists, however, make a distinction between the two terms that is important to successful therapy.

Fear is a basic, automatic response to a specific object, situation, or circumstance that involves a recognition (perception) of actual or potential danger.[4] For someone with arachnophobia, anything that suggests the possible presence of a spider, such as a spider's web, an older house, walking in the forest, even a picture of a spider, might elicit fear. Whenever outside, this person might be constantly thinking, "I wonder whether I will come across a spider," "Spiders are dangerous because they can crawl into your mouth or ears and lay eggs," or "If I see a spider, I'll freak out." Physically, this person might feel tense, on edge, have butterflies in the stomach, chest tightness, or a racing heart whenever he sees something that reminds him of spiders. And the fear could cause a change in behavior, such as avoiding any places thought to risk exposure to spiders. In terms of cognitive therapy, the main characteristic of fear is *a thought of imminent threat or danger to one's safety.*

> Fear is a basic, automatic state of alarm consisting of a perception or conclusion of imminent threat or danger to your safety and security.[5]

Anxiety, in contrast, is a much more prolonged, complex emotional state that is often triggered by an initial fear. For example, you could feel anxious about going to visit friends because they live in an older home that might have spiders or about going to the movies because the film might contain a scene with spiders. The basic fear is of encountering a spider, but you live in a state of persistent anxiety about the *future possibility* of being exposed to a spider. So anxiety is a more enduring experience than fear. It's a *state* of apprehension and physical arousal in which you believe you can't control or pre-

> Anxiety is a prolonged, complex emotional state that occurs when a person anticipates that some future situation, event, or circumstance may involve a personally distressing, unpredictable, and uncontrollable threat to his or her vital interests.

dict potentially aversive future events. Thus you might feel anxious thinking about an important interview, going to a dinner party where you don't know people, traveling to an unfamiliar place, your performance at work, or a deadline. Notice that anxiety is always future oriented; it is driven by "what if?" thinking. We don't become anxious over the past, what has already happened; rather, we become anxious over *imagined future adverse events or catastrophes:* "What if my mind goes blank during the exam?" "What if I don't get all my work done?" "What if I have a panic attack in the supermarket?" "What if I get the H1N1 influenza virus by being around people?" "What if I encounter someone who reminds me of the assailant who attacked me?" "What if I lose my job?" This enduring emotional state that we call anxiety is the focus of this workbook.

How Do Fear and Anxiety Operate Together?

Fear is at the heart of all anxiety states. When we're anxious, fear is the underlying psychological state that drives the anxiety. Jan has social anxiety. Whenever she even thinks about going to a meeting, she becomes intensely anxious. However, the fear underlying her anxiety is embarrassment: "What if I'm asked a question I can't answer? Everyone will think I'm incompetent, and I'll feel unbearably embarrassed." Larry has health anxiety. Whenever he has the slightest feeling of abdominal upset, he feels anxious. His underlying, or core, fear is "What if I get terribly sick, start vomiting, can't stop, and suffocate from not being able to breathe?" Mary has agoraphobia. Whenever she thinks about going to the supermarket, she gets anxious. Her underlying fear is that she will have a severe panic attack in the supermarket: "What if I make a big scene in front of all those people?" Mack also has agoraphobia. He feels anxious even thinking about driving across a suspension bridge. His underlying fear is that he'll be so tense while driving that he'll lose control of the car and drive over the side.

Cognitive therapy, and the work you'll do in this workbook, focuses on the fear at the core of your anxiety, so it's important to have a firm grasp of the fear that underlies your anxiety experiences. See if you can identify that core fear using Worksheet 2.1. If you're working with a therapist, no doubt you will be spending time identifying the core fear that underlies your anxiety state.

⋛ Troubleshooting Tips ⋚

You may be having difficulty identifying the core fear that occurs when you feel anxious, because most of us focus on the feelings of anxiety more than on what is making us anxious. Ask yourself "What is so threatening or upsetting about this situation?" and "What's so bad about this situation?" Sometimes the core fear in anxiety is simply the fear that you'll feel anxious. If you're still having trouble filling in Worksheet 2.1, read further into the chapter and then come back to it later.

Unraveling Anxiety

Part of the definition of anxiety is that it's complex. When you feel highly anxious, you're affected physically, emotionally, behaviorally, and, of course, cognitively.

To use cognitive therapy strategies effectively to reduce anxiety, it's important to discover the core fear, your evaluation of threat, that lies behind your anxiety episodes.

You might not always be aware of it at the time you're anxious, but in an anxious state you think, feel, and behave differently than when you're not anxious. Here are some of the common effects of anxiety:

Physical Symptoms

- Increased heart rate, palpitations
- Shortness of breath, rapid breathing
- Chest pain or pressure
- Choking sensation
- Dizziness, lightheadedness
- Sweating, hot flashes, chills

Discovering the Core Fear Behind Your Anxiety

Anxiety State	Core Fear
Briefly describe what makes you feel anxious. What situations or events trigger your anxiety? When are you most likely to feel anxious? What might you avoid doing because you would feel too anxious?	Try to identify the core fear behind your anxiety. What is the worst that could happen in the anxious situation? Is there some catastrophic outcome you fear? What is the threat or danger posed to you or your loved ones?
1.	1.
2.	2.
3.	3.
4.	4.
5.	5.

- Nausea, upset stomach, diarrhea
- Trembling, shaking
- Tingling or numbness in arms, legs
- Weakness, unsteadiness, faintness
- Tense muscles, rigidity
- Dry mouth

Cognitive Symptoms

- Fear of losing control, being unable to cope
- Fear of physical injury or death
- Fear of "going crazy"
- Fear of negative evaluation by others
- Frightening thoughts, images, or memories
- Perceptions of unreality or detachment
- Poor concentration, confusion, distractibility
- Narrowing of attention, hypervigilance for threat
- Poor memory
- Difficulty in reasoning, loss of objectivity

Behavioral Symptoms

- Avoidance of threat cues or situations
- Escape, flight
- Pursuit of safety, reassurance
- Restlessness, agitation, pacing
- Hyperventilation
- Freezing, motionlessness
- Difficulty speaking

Emotional Symptoms

- Feeling nervous, tense, wound up
- Feeling frightened, fearful, terrified
- Being edgy, jumpy, jittery
- Being impatient, frustrated

Think back to a recent anxiety episode. If you run through the preceding lists, can you identify the physical, cognitive, behavioral, and emotional symptoms that occur when you feel anxious? Rebecca is anxious about having to confront an employee who repeatedly arrives late for work. Her core fear is that he will get angry and there will be a confrontation. A fear of confrontation underlies much of the anxiety Rebecca feels when having to be assertive with employees. When she wakes up in the morning, her anxiety is triggered by remembering that today she has to confront Dave, her employee, about his tardiness. She immediately notices certain physical symptoms like an elevated heart rate and tight neck muscles and emotional symptoms like a general sense of being jittery and keyed up. As she gets ready for work, her cognitive symptoms include thinking about all the things that could go wrong during their conversation: "What if I make a fool of myself in front of Dave because I'll be shaking and he'll notice I'm anxious and think he can walk all over me?" "What if I end up 'caving in' and just tell him to try to do better—which, of course, will mean that he'll just keep on doing what he's doing?" "What if he gets angry or defensive and starts yelling at me?" "What if he goes around bad-mouthing me to the rest of the department?" By the time Rebecca climbs into her car, she's irritable and ends up honking at everyone who doesn't drive exactly the way she wants. She's distracted and almost misses her turn as she rehearses what she'll say over and over once she finally sees Dave. The behavioral symptom of avoidance kicks in as soon as she gets to work, with Rebecca thinking of several priorities that seem more important than talking to Dave. Later in the morning he sends her an e-mail, which she ignores (again avoidance) even though she knows responding would give her the perfect opportunity to ask him to come to her office. By the end of the day she feels the emotional symptoms of frustration and anger at herself, at Dave, and, when she gets home, at her husband and children because once again she has procrastinated in dealing with an important personnel problem at work.

Worksheet 2.2 is a form you can use to fill in the symptoms of your own anxiety for different anxious concerns. Look at the example filled out for Rebecca that follows the worksheet. The first concern filled out in Rebecca's worksheet is the one just described.

It's natural to feel overwhelmed by anxiety. Breaking down your anxiety experiences and dealing with each component will make anxiety feel less intimidating. Once you understand the components of your anxiety, you'll be ready to apply the cognitive therapy strategies to them.

To fill out your own worksheet, focus on two or three typical anxiety episodes that you have recently experienced—a recent period of intense worry, a panic attack, a feeling of intense anxiety. Describe the anxiety episode or concern in the left column and then break it down into physical, cognitive, behavioral, and emotional symptoms. You can refer to the lists of symptoms on pages 16 and 18 for some ideas. If you can't remember a past anxiety episode well enough to do the exercise, try to fill in the form the next time you have an

Your Anxiety Symptoms

Anxious Concern (What are you feeling anxious about?)	Physical Symptoms (When anxious, what physical sensations do you experience?)	Cognitive Symptoms (What goes through your mind when you are anxious? What are you thinking about?)	Behavioral Symptoms (How do you behave when anxious? What do you do?)	Affective Symptoms (How do you feel when anxious?)
1.				
2.				
3.				

Rebecca's Anxiety Symptoms

Anxious Concern (What are you feeling anxious about?)	Physical Symptoms (When anxious, what physical sensations do you experience?)	Cognitive Symptoms (What goes through your mind when you are anxious? What are you thinking about?)	Behavioral Symptoms (How do you behave when anxious? What do you do?)	Affective Symptoms (How do you feel when anxious?)
1. Thinking about need to confront a tardy employee	Chest pressure, weakness, lightheaded, rapid heart rate, tension	What if the employee gets angry and we have a confrontation? What if he notices I'm anxious and thinks I'm weak? What if I'm not assertive enough? What if he talks behind my back and the employees lose respect for me?	I rehearse over and over what to say; procrastinate, avoid the employee.	Nervous, tense, impatient, frustrated
2. Thinking about my parents being disappointed that I haven't visited them recently	Tense muscles	I should take the time to visit them more. I am being such a bad daughter. What if one of them passes away? Then I'll be sorry I didn't visit more. How can I find the time when I'm so busy at work and home?	I avoid talking to my parents; make promises to visit them next week.	Frustrated, depressed, on edge, tense
3. Looking over the monthly bills	Tight chest, lightheaded, weakness, tense muscles, a little shaky	How will we pay all these bills? Our spending is out of control; we'll end up having to declare bankruptcy. [I experience poor concentration, confusion, can't think through to a solution.]	I avoid opening the monthly bills; procrastinate making bill payments; continue to spend.	Frustrated, irritable, discouraged, nervous

anxiety episode. If you are using the workbook as a therapy companion, being aware of the different components of your anxiety episodes will help you collaborate with your therapist in developing a treatment plan.

"Should I Work On My Anxiety?"

You may already know from your own experience that anxiety ranges in severity, not only from person to person but also in the same person, from episode to episode. The fact that "it's not always that bad" may in fact be the reason you haven't addressed your own anxiety before now. And you may still wonder whether you should bother, especially if you're not already seeing a therapist. In Chapter 1 we asked you to write down why you want your experience of anxiety to change and what your goals are. These insights can be important motivators. So can understanding where your anxiety experience falls on the continuum from mild to severe. Taking a good look at how big a problem anxiety is in your life can provide the impetus you need to work through this book, with or without professional help.

It can be very difficult to judge for yourself what's "normal" or "abnormal" anxiety. This is where a thorough evaluation by a trained mental health professional can give you perspective. Every time a mental health professional sees a new client with anxiety, he or she must determine whether the client is suffering an anxiety disorder, the severity of the anxiety, and the degree of interference in daily living caused by the condition. If your anxiety is severe and qualifies as a disorder, it might be particularly important to seek a more formal treatment intervention from a trained professional. However, you can still use the workbook strategies and incorporate them into the therapy sessions for your anxiety disorder.

Mental health practitioners use a textbook published by the American Psychiatric Association to determine whether a person meets the diagnostic criteria for an anxiety disorder. Called the *Diagnostic and Statistical Manual of Mental Disorders, Fourth Edition, Text Revision* (DSM-IV-TR),[14] it provides a well-defined set of criteria for many types of anxiety disorders as well as hundreds of other mental and emotional disturbances. However, even with a diagnostic manual, determining whether a person has an anxiety disorder can be difficult, because we have no physical test for anxiety. So the assessment must depend on self-reported symptoms; these symptoms often change over time and across situations, and people differ in how well they tolerate anxiety. In our practice we have seen people who have lived with intense levels of anxiety on a daily basis and yet only reluctantly sought treatment after many years.

Despite these uncertainties, there are specific characteristics that therapists assess when making a diagnosis of anxiety. How many of these characteristics you have, and to what extent, will determine whether a therapist would diagnose you with an anxiety disorder. Even if you don't have a disorder, you may benefit from receiving some form of professional help, but having a disorder means that you should seriously consider whether to seek more formal treatment from a qualified mental health professional. Therapists use several characteristics to determine whether a person's anxiety qualifies as a clinical disorder:

1. **Exaggerated intensity.** Clinical anxiety tends to be much greater than one would expect in a particular situation. For example, experiencing intense anxiety when answering the phone, driving across a bridge, making a request of a store clerk, or touching a doorknob would suggest an abnormal level of anxiety because these types of actions cause little or no anxiety for most people.

2. **Persistence.** Clinical anxiety tends to persist longer than nonclinical states. Everyone worries from time to time, but people with pathological worry experience it for hours, day in and day out.

3. **Interference.** Clinical anxiety tends to interfere with functioning at work or school, social events, recreation, family relations, and other routine activities. The negative effects of anxiety may be limited to certain areas of life, but the impact is definitely noticeable. Some individuals with agoraphobia, for example, will do their grocery shopping at 3:00 A.M. to avoid other people; others will drive many extra miles in traffic to avoid crossing a certain bridge; and people with generalized anxiety may not be able to fall asleep at night because of worry.

4. **Sudden anxiety or panic.** An occasional surge of anxiety or even panic isn't uncommon, but frequent occurrences may represent an anxiety disorder. Spontaneous, "out of the blue" panic is particularly noteworthy, and developing a fear of having further panic attacks is a significant feature of anxiety disorders. (For further discussion of panic attacks, see Chapter 9.)

5. **Generalization.** In anxiety disorders, the fear and anxiety often spread from a particular object or situation to a broad range of situations, tasks, objects, or people. Mary, for example, had her first panic attack while in a crowded restaurant. It really scared her, so she started checking to make sure restaurants weren't too crowded before entering. This progressed to selecting only less popular restaurants and going at off hours. Eventually Mary stopped going to restaurants and other public places altogether, for fear that she might get that "trapped feeling" and begin to feel anxious. Mary's anxiety was spreading, causing greater interference and limitations in her life.

6. **Catastrophic thinking.** People with clinical anxiety tend to think about worst-case scenarios. Because anxiety always involves the anticipated (the "what ifs"), the thinking style in anxiety disorders is biased toward assuming that serious threats are much more likely than they actually are. For example, a person with panic disorder might automatically think, "I'm having trouble catching my breath. What if I suffocate to death?" Someone with social anxiety thinks,

"What if people notice that I'm nervous and wonder if I am mentally ill?" A person with generalized anxiety might think, "If I don't stop worrying, it will drive me crazy." All of this thinking involves the possibility ("what ifs") of some catastrophe that is an exaggeration of the real danger. Chapter 3 focuses exclusively on how anxiety changes our way of thinking.

7. **Avoidance.** Most people with anxiety disorders try to eliminate or at least minimize their anxiety by avoiding anything that triggers it. Triggers could be certain situations (e.g., crowded stores, highway driving, public facilities, meetings, movie theaters, or church), people (unfamiliar people, "sketchy" individuals, people in authority, ill people, etc.), or objects (such as bridges, tunnels, hospitals, certain animals). Extensive avoidance might reduce anxiety in the short term, but it comes at a high cost. It contributes to persistence of the anxiety condition and reduces a person's level of daily functioning. The problem of avoidance is discussed more thoroughly in Chapter 7.

8. **Loss of safety or feeling calm.** Finally, individuals with an anxiety disorder often feel less safe or secure than others. Although they may go to great lengths to feel safe, any sense of security is short lived, and the feeling of apprehension and threat returns. Relaxing or staying calm can be quite difficult. In anxiety disorders the person may feel on edge, keyed up, and agitated more often than not. Difficulty sleeping can be a major problem in most of the anxiety disorders.

If you're not currently working with a professional, or you are still in the assessment phase of therapy, fill in Worksheet 2.3, an Anxiety Disorder Checklist that we've developed to help you get an idea of whether you may have clinical anxiety. Only a qualified professional can provide an accurate diagnosis, but if you answer "yes" to most of the statements on the checklist, you should consider seeking professional help. This workbook was written for people with anxiety disorders, so it should help you whether you are seeing a professional and whether your anxiety qualifies as a disorder or is subclinical. If you are currently in therapy, discuss your answers to the checklist questions with your therapist. She may want you to elaborate on your responses, especially if therapy is still in the assessment phase.

The Many Faces of Anxiety Disorders

Not all anxiety disorders are the same. DSM-IV-TR[14] lists 13 different types of anxiety disorders (Martin Antony and Peter Norton provide a very concise and informative description of all 13 anxiety disorders in their self-help book *The Anti-Anxiety Workbook*[15]). Our workbook focuses on three anxiety disorders—panic disorder with or without agoraphobia, social phobia, and generalized anxiety disorder (GAD).

The Anxiety Disorder Checklist

Instructions: This checklist consists of a series of statements about anxiety. Place a checkmark in the "yes" or "no" box to indicate whether the statement describes your experience of anxiety. If you find that most of the statements apply to your anxiety, consider whether you are experiencing clinically significant anxiety and should seek professional help if you're not already working with a therapist.

Item	Yes	No
1. My anxiety episodes are moderately to severely distressing to me.		
2. I am anxious about ordinary, everyday situations or tasks that most people face without difficulty.		
3. I have anxiety episodes daily or at least several times a week.		
4. I have had problems with anxiety for several months or even years.		
5. My anxiety episodes last longer than would be expected, given the situation.		
6. I avoid certain places, situations, people, or activities because of anxiety.		
7. Anxiety interferes in my work (school), relationships with people, and/or family relations.		
8. I tend to catastrophize (think of the worst outcome) when anxious.		
9. I experience sudden onsets of anxiety or panic attacks.		
10. My anxiety has spread so it now includes a number of different situations, objects, people, tasks, and so forth.		
11. I am not very successful at controlling anxiety without medication.		
12. I have become quite fearful of the anxiety episodes.		
13. It is increasingly difficult to feel calm or safe.		
14. Close friends or family members think I have an anxiety problem.		
15. I have always tended to be an anxious or nervous person.		

These are among the most common mental health conditions and represent complex emotional states. They also often occur together in the same person. People with panic disorder often feel anxious in social situations, for example, so you may benefit from working on more than one of the specialized chapters (Chapters 9–11). Specific cognitive therapy protocols have been developed for each of these disorders. Although obsessive–compulsive disorder (OCD) and posttraumatic stress disorder (PTSD) are covered in our professional therapy book,[5] they are not included here because the core fear and manifestations of OCD and PTSD differ somewhat from those of other anxiety disorders. We do, however, list resources for all five anxiety disorders at the back of this book.

Table 2.1 summarizes the core features of the three anxiety disorders covered in this workbook, focusing on the situations or concerns that uniquely trigger anxiety in each disorder and the typical thought process that characterizes it. More complete symptom descriptions of the disorders can be found in Chapters 9–11.

Whether or not you have an anxiety disorder, the individual symptoms of anxiety need to change. Therefore this workbook targets the symptoms of anxiety disorders, outlined in Table 2.1, and whatever types of anxiety problems you experience, you should find the cognitive and behavioral strategies in this workbook useful for achieving meaningful reductions in your symptoms. The specialized chapters may also have relevance for you, regardless of your diagnosis, because they target major anxiety symptoms like panic attacks (Chapter 9), social anxiety (Chapter 10), and worry (Chapter 11). Using the strategies of cognitive therapy, you have every reason to expect anxiety to play a less intrusive role in your life. In other words, things are about to get a lot better.

TABLE 2.1. Summary Description of Three Common Anxiety Disorders

Anxiety disorder	Anxiety trigger	Fearful (catastrophic) thinking
Panic disorder (with or without agoraphobia)	Physical, bodily sensations (e.g., having heart palpitations, breathlessness, lightheaded)	Fear of dying ("heart attack"), losing control ("going crazy") or consciousness (fainting), having further panic attacks
Generalized anxiety disorder (GAD)	Stressful life events or other personal concerns	Fear of possible future adverse or threatening life outcomes
Social phobia	Social, public situations; exposure to other people's attention	Fear of negative evaluation from others (e.g., embarrassment, humiliation)

Note. Reprinted with permission from *Cognitive Therapy of Anxiety Disorders* by David A. Clark and Aaron T. Beck (p. 9). Copyright 2010 by The Guilford Press.

CHAPTER SUMMARY

- Fear is the perception (i.e., thought) of imminent threat or danger to an individual's safety or security.

- Fear is at the root of anxiety, and so discovering the core fear that drives anxiety is important in cognitive therapy.

- Anxiety is a more enduring emotional state that occurs when individuals anticipate a personally aversive, unpredictable, and uncontrollable future situation that is perceived to threaten their vital interests.

- To understand anxiety you need to know its symptoms or how it is expressed in the physical, cognitive, behavioral, and emotional domains.

- There is no clear boundary between normal and abnormal anxiety states. However, clinical anxiety (i.e., a disorder) tends to be more exaggerated, unrealistic, intense, persistent, generalized, and interfering in daily living than nonclinical anxiety states.

- There are many different types of anxiety disorders. This workbook focuses on three of the most common; panic disorder (including agoraphobia), social anxiety, and generalized anxiety (including worry).

Earlier we explained that the main characteristic of fear is the *thought* of imminent threat or danger and that fear is at the heart of all anxiety states. That's why *cognitive* therapy is so effective in treating anxiety—and why it's important to understand the workings of the anxious mind, the subject of the next chapter.

3

The Anxious Mind

A few years ago my (D. A. C.) youngest daughter, Christina, turned 16, and, like most Canadian and American youth, she was keen on learning to drive. We enrolled her in a driver education course, and she progressed through the various stages of the program. Upon completion she successfully passed the written exam and was given a learner's permit. She immediately started asking me to take her driving. I agreed, and so the day arrived when Christina and I headed for a lonely country road in our county. I drove to our destination, pulled the car over to the side of the road, and said to Christina, "Okay, you take the wheel now." Her anxiety during that entire drive to the country was obvious (my anxiety began after she took the wheel!). I recall her squeezing the steering wheel, every muscle in her body tense. She stared intently at the road ahead and screamed when she met her first oncoming vehicle (it was a two-lane country road). Our car slowed to a crawl until the other car passed.

Over the next 15 minutes, Christina and I showed all the classic signs of high anxiety. But by the end of our driving expedition (30 minutes), our anxiety level had dropped significantly. Over the next several days we took many driving tours, and each time our anxiety level was a little less intense and became briefer and briefer. Finally, after 2 weeks of driving in the country, Christina showed no signs of anxiety. However, when we subsequently switched to city driving, the same scenario started all over again, with initially high anxiety followed by declining levels of intensity with repeated practice.

There are two facts about anxiety we can learn from this story of the brief life of an anxious moment:

- *Anxiety declines naturally if left alone.*
- *Anxiety varies greatly between situations and from person to person.*

You may immediately disagree with this conclusion. You may be thinking, "That's not true for me; I'm anxious almost daily, and it lasts for hours," or "Anyone would be anxious if he had to go through what I experience." We're not suggesting that all anxiety experiences are brief or that some situations would not make most people anxious. Instead we pose a different question:

If anxiety declines naturally, how do we turn it into a persistent state?

Let's look at the driving example to illustrate the situation.

Christina's anxiety over driving declined quite rapidly with repeated experience. But what would have to happen for Christina's anxiety to remain elevated? To remain highly anxious she would have to be preoccupied with thoughts like these:

■ *Driving is dangerous* ("I could so easily have an accident," "I could get seriously injured or killed," "Many young, inexperienced drivers have accidents," "Maybe other drivers are not paying attention to the road").

■ *I'm a terrible driver and will never be able to learn to drive* ("I don't know what I am doing," "I can't remember all the driving information," "What if I step on the gas pedal instead of the brake?", "I'm so anxious I know I'll make a terrible driver," "I'm so poorly coordinated, I can't imagine how I could become a confident driver").

■ *Better to remain safe and avoid driving* ("I won't feel this terrible anxiety if I avoid learning to drive," "It's safer if I'm a passenger and leave the driving to someone with more experience," "Being able to drive is not necessary for survival").

■ *Being so worried means driving must be dangerous* ("What if I have an accident and wreck the car?", "What if I remain overly nervous every time I get behind the wheel?", "If I don't learn to relax while driving, I might be more likely to have an accident").

When Christina's anxiety actually declined with repeated driving experiences, what was she thinking?

■ *Driving is an acceptable risk* ("Relative to the number of drivers on the road, accidents are not that common," "I'm on a lonely country road, which is pretty safe," "I'm driving so slowly, it's hard to believe I could get hurt if I did something wrong," "My father can grab the steering wheel if I make a mistake").

■ *I can learn to drive* ("Everyone has to start out as a learner; if they can do it, I can too," "I've got pretty good coordination skills," "I'm paying very close attention to the road," "I'm driving as cautiously as one can").

■ *Better to overcome my fears now* ("I'm confident my anxiety will decrease the more I practice driving," "If I don't face my anxiety about driving now, it will only get worse later," "If I don't learn to drive, I'll remain forever dependent on others").

■ *I need to remain problem focused* ("I've been anxious before when learning a new skill and was able to overcome my reluctance," "I need to concentrate on what I learned in my driving lessons; I've got all the necessary information to be an effective driver").

The important point is that **the way you think determines whether anxiety persists or declines.** Thinking about threat or danger ("driving kills") and vulnerability or helplessness ("I can't do this") will cause anxiety to persist. Thinking about acceptable risk ("Driving is an acceptable risk that millions take daily in our society") and personal ability ("I can deal with this situation") leads to a decline in anxiety.

This chapter is a foundation for the entire workbook. It explains that how we think can cause anxiety to persist and make us unable to turn it off. Understanding the cognitive (thinking) basis of your anxiety is a critical first step in cognitive therapy for anxiety. You will want to return to this chapter frequently as you read subsequent chapters in the workbook. As you read through this chapter, try to apply the explanations and concepts to your experience of anxiety.

Thinking Dangerously

Imagine you were asked to walk across a board that is 6 inches wide, 8 feet long, and 1 foot off the ground. Could you do it? Would you feel afraid? I doubt you would feel any fear, and, yes, you could probably easily walk the board as long as you had normal balance. But what if we move the board so it is 50 feet off the ground? Would you walk across it now? My guess is that most people would say "No, thank you." Would you feel afraid, nervous? Most of us would say "You bet."

So why the different feelings and response to the same task, walking a 6-inch-wide board? The answer lies in how we think about danger. Most people would think walking a board 50 feet off the ground too dangerous: "If I lose my balance, I could fall to my death," "I probably would lose my balance because the height would make me feel dizzy," "This is silly—it's just not worth the risk." Maybe an acrobat would not be anxious because she would think "This is not dangerous; I've done this hundreds of times." On the other hand, most people would not view walking a board that's only 1 foot off the ground as dangerous.

In the last couple of decades, hundreds of experimental studies have found that people become overly focused on threat and danger when anxious.[5,16,17] Also thoughts, images, or memories of personal threat or danger can cause people to feel fear or anxiety.

The problem in anxiety disorders is that people tend to overestimate both the likelihood and the intensity of threat and danger.

■ Do you find yourself often thinking that a threat or danger is **very likely** to happen to you or loved ones (e.g., that you *probably* will mess up the interview, that you *probably* will embarrass yourself, that *probably* there is something wrong with you)?

■ Do you find yourself often thinking that the **worst will happen** (that you will *never* get a promotion, that *everyone* will think you're an idiot, that you won't be able to catch your breath and will *suffocate to death,* that you will contract a *deadly disease*)?

We call this type of dangerous thinking *catastrophizing,* or blowing things out of proportion.[18] When we are anxious, we tend to catastrophize about the ordinary, everyday experiences of life; we think the worst-case scenario is much more likely to occur than it is. Overestimating the likelihood and severity of threat is a key feature of the core fear underlying anxiety that you read about in Chapter 2. Therefore catching and correcting your catastrophic thinking is an important cognitive therapy strategy for reducing fear and anxiety. Table 3.1 illustrates some common experiences that individuals with anxiety tend to catastrophize.

Most of the things listed in Table 3.1 are ordinary experiences, but in anxiety we tend to interpret these events as threatening by engaging in dangerous thinking (catastrophizing): we tend to overestimate, exaggerate, or be unrealistic about the likelihood that the worst-case scenario (the catastrophe) will occur.

Try completing Worksheet 3.1 to see if you can capture how you might be thinking too dangerously, or catastrophizing, during your anxiety episodes. Catastrophic thinking tends to happen very quickly and automatically when we're anxious, so you might have difficulty coming up with your anxious thoughts. If you're reading this workbook on your own, try identifying the triggers and then, when you encounter these situations, try to catch your thinking while in that situation. If you still have trouble completing the worksheet, you can return to it after you've finished the chapter.

⌇ Troubleshooting Tips ⌇

Most people find it difficult to catch their anxious thinking because they tend to be overly focused on how bad they feel. If you're working with a therapist, identifying anxious thoughts will be a skill you'll work on in therapy. If you are reading this workbook on your own, you can wait until your anxiety has settled down before you fill in Worksheet 3.1. Then ask yourself, "What did I think was the worst possible thing that could happen to me dur-

TABLE 3.1. **Common Examples of Catastrophizing in Anxiety Disorders**

Anxious concern (trigger)	Overestimated probability	Overestimated severity (worst-case scenario)
1. Feeling anxious about going to movies with a friend	"It will be crowded, we'll have to sit in the center of the row, and I'll be anxious."	"I'll have a panic attack in the middle of the movie; I won't be able to get out, and I'll be 'freaking out'; it will be the worst panic I've had in a while."
2. Feeling anxious about unexpected interview with boss	"I'm going to be told that my work is not satisfactory; I'll probably be very nervous, hot, and uncomfortable."	"I'm going to lose my job; at the very least I'll be so anxious and panicky that my boss will wonder what's wrong with me."
3. Feeling anxious about mailing my tax return	"I will probably get audited and have to pay a lot of extra income tax."	"The audit will result in a substantial tax bill. I'm already 'maxed out' on my line of credit and won't be able to pay it. I'll have to declare bankruptcy."
4. Feeling anxious whenever I have the thought that I could die young	"I wonder if having these disturbing thoughts that I could die young means that I will die at a young age."	"What a terrible tragedy to die in my twenties and never get to live a full life; to miss out on all the things that other people experience."
5. Feeling anxious because I can't get to sleep due to worry	"I'll never get to sleep. I'll never be able to control this worry and sleep normally again."	"My life is completely ruined by not being able to sleep. My concentration at work is so poor, I'm sure I'll be fired."
6. Feeling anxious about chest pain	"I shouldn't be having these chest pains now. There must be something wrong with my heart."	"I could be having a heart attack. I am too far from the hospital. Doctors will get to me too late, and so I'll die from this heart attack."

ing that anxiety episode?" and "What scared me about this situation?" or "What was so upsetting about this situation?" If you still can't think of possible cognitions you had when feeling anxious, ask someone you know who also might be even a little anxious in a similar situation what he or she thinks about. This might help bring up some ideas for you on what you may be thinking in that situation.

Your "Dangerous Thinking" Profile When Feeling Anxious

Anxious Concern Briefly describe the situation that triggers the anxious experience. What has made you feel anxious?	Overestimated Probability What is the negative outcome of the anxious experience? What are you thinking is the likelihood of this negative outcome?	Overestimated Severity What is the worst-case outcome in this situation? What is the catastrophe that has crossed your mind? How bad could it get?
1.		
2.		
3.		
4.		
5.		

Why Is Catastrophic Thinking So Easy?

The core fear that underlies anxiety involves a tendency to automatically think dangerously—to catastrophize—exaggerating the probability and severity of bad outcomes of common, everyday situations.

If you're thinking that you know you tend to assume the worst when anxious but can't stop yourself—or that anxiety comes on so quickly that you're not aware of anything going through your mind—you're not alone. Over the last two decades, psychologists have learned a great deal about anxious thinking. We now know that anxious thinking happens very quickly (in less than half a second!) and automatically so that people are not even aware their brain is processing threat and danger. Also, when those who suffer from anxiety disorders anticipate a situation that typically makes them feel anxious, their brain automatically scans the environment for signs of threat—what we call *danger cues*. Even our memory system and reasoning abilities become biased when we are anxious so that we tend to recall past anxious or frightening experiences and generate threatening explanations and expectations. In other words, our whole mental system becomes locked into an anxious mind-set. This all occurs automatically, rapidly, and involuntarily. You don't have to think "Oh, let me see, it's time to think anxiously." Instead you are thinking anxiously before you realize it.

Cognitive therapy was developed to help you learn how to override or shut down this anxious mind-set. To use a computer analogy, in anxiety disorders the dangerous mind-set is like a software virus that invades your operating system. Cognitive therapy teaches you how to detect and override the catastrophizing virus so it no longer has complete control over how you think. **Change the way you think to change the way you feel.** Anxiety reduction will occur once "dangerous thinking" has been shut down.

Cognitive therapy strategies can teach you how to detect and override exaggerated, automatic thoughts of threat and danger.

"But I Feel So Helpless"

It's hard to believe in yourself—believe you can handle a situation effectively—when you're feeling anxious about it. When we feel afraid or anxious, we also tend to see ourselves as weak, vulnerable, and unable to cope. So along with the automatic threat or danger thoughts, when anxious you may feel helpless and unable to cope. However, these thoughts are a slower, more effortful response to a perceived threat than catastrophizing. Therefore you may be more aware of thinking you're helpless than of your more automatic catastrophic thoughts.

You may feel helpless because you believe you lack the skills necessary to deal with the anxious situation. Self-doubt and a profound sense of uncertainty will intensify your sense of vulnerability. The problem with vulnerability thinking in anxiety is that it usually involves a distortion of reality; you're not as weak and unable to cope with the situation as you think. The relation of danger (anxiety) and vulnerability (helplessness) thinking to anxiety can be expressed in the following formula:

Overestimate Danger + Underestimate Personal Coping = High Anxiety

Each of the people introduced in Chapter 1 had automatic threat and personal vulnerability thoughts. When Rebecca worried about work, she thought about her employees losing respect for her (dangerous thinking) and about not being able to confront her employees effectively (helplessness thinking). Todd would have unexpected heart palpitations and then worry it might be a heart attack (dangerous thinking) and he wouldn't get to the hospital in time (helplessness thinking). Elizabeth worried about embarrassing herself in front of other people (dangerous thinking) and not being able to carry on a coherent conversation (helplessness thinking).

When you're feeling anxious, what types of helpless thoughts run through your mind? See how well you can capture these thoughts by completing Worksheet 3.2. Record the anxious experience in the first column and then in the second column describe how you feel weak and vulnerable in the situation. How would you respond in the situation that might be unhelpful in the long run? How might you behave or attempt to cope in a way that would increase the perceived threat and make the anxiety worse? In the final column, describe what you think would be the ideal, most effective way to cope with the anxious situation. How would you like to respond that would be a strong, confident response to the situation?

In addition to changing automatic thoughts about threat and danger, cognitive therapy works on changing how you see yourself in anxious situations. In cognitive therapy we help the anxious person evaluate and correct her vulnerability thoughts and beliefs so she has greater self-confidence to deal with anxious concerns. Your responses to Worksheet 3.2 therefore play an important role in our approach to anxiety reduction. In fact, you'll use this worksheet to fill out your own personal Anxiety Profile in Chapter 5.

⋛ Troubleshooting Tips ⋚

If you're having difficulty identifying your anxiety helplessness thoughts, ask yourself, "When I'm anxious, do I feel like I've lost control? If so, how have I lost control over my body (physical), over my emotions, over my thinking, and over my behavior?" How you think about loss of control when anxious is a good way to identify your helplessness cognitions. If you're in therapy, you can discuss Worksheet 3.2 with your therapist to be clearer on how you underestimate your ability to cope with anxious situations.

Your "Helpless Thinking" Profile When Feeling Anxious

Anxious Concern Briefly describe the situation that triggers the anxious experience. What has made you feel anxious?	Helplessness Thinking How are you acting weak or helpless in this situation? How are you overwhelmed by the situation? How do you end up responding, coping? What do you expect of yourself in this situation?	Desired Coping Response How would you like to respond to this situation? What would be a strong, confident way of coping? What is the most effective way to cope with this anxious concern? Do you have someone in mind who copes so well with these situations?
1.		
2.		
3.		
4.		
5.		

Dangerous Errors

Think back to the last time you were really anxious. Did it involve an uncomfortable situation like being around unfamiliar people or in an unfamiliar place, sitting in a hot and crowded room, or the like? Did you find that

> Cognitive therapy focuses on strengthening your self-confidence and ability to cope with anxious situations.

all you could think about was how bad you were feeling and how much you wanted to get out of the situation? Did you notice that you became entirely focused on your anxiety and couldn't seem to concentrate on anything else around you? Anxiety does this; it distorts our thinking process so that we become narrowly focused on threat, danger, and helplessness.

This narrowed thinking is extremely important to our survival when real danger exists. If someone approaches you on the street who looks threatening to you, your full attention needs to be on figuring out whether this person is going to mug you or is harmless. No time to be looking at store windows, checking your phone, or planning the evening meal. You need to make a very quick decision and identify a quick escape route.

But what happens when there is no external danger? When the danger is merely anticipated—a thought and not an actual event, such as "What if I am getting sick?" or "What if I have a panic attack?" or "What if I make a mistake?"—your anxious thinking is, unfortunately, still selective. When anxious, you're not likely to be aware of this narrowing, but how you see reality is in fact distorted. Table 3.2 lists a number of thinking "errors" that result from this distortion when people feel anxious. Read through the definitions and examples, checking off the ones that seem most relevant to you. You'll use this information later in the book.

When these thinking errors focus your attention exclusively on threat and danger, *they make it impossible for you to consider less threatening or benign interpretations of situations.* **This exclusion prolongs the experience of anxiety.**

Have you ever noticed how hard it is to focus on aspects of a situation that suggest it is safer and less threatening than you think? In the midst of anxiety it's very difficult to think rationally or constructively. Whenever Janet started worrying about her work performance and whether her supervisor thought she was competent, she

> Cognitive therapy can teach you to become more aware of the cognitive errors that characterize your anxious thinking so you can question your anxious thoughts and shift to a more constructive perspective on your anxious concerns.

couldn't make herself think about her past successes or remember that she had never had any indication that she was perceived as incompetent. Because of jumping to conclusions, tunnel vision, catastrophizing, and other cognitive distortions, Janet's thought processes became locked on to the danger thoughts ("My supervisor will think I'm incompetent"). The same thing happened to Pierre when he had unexpected chest pains and

TABLE 3.2. Thinking Errors That Are Common in Anxiety

The following is a list of thinking errors that are common when people feel afraid or anxious. You may find that you make some of these errors when you feel anxious, but you probably don't make all of the errors every time you are anxious. Read through the list of errors with their definition and examples. Put a check mark beside the ones that are particularly relevant for you. You will notice the errors overlap because they all deal with different aspects of overestimating threat and underestimating your coping ability and safety when feeling anxious.

Thinking error	Definition	Examples
Catastrophizing (overestimating threat and danger)	Focusing on the worst possible outcome in an anxious situation	• Thinking that chest tightness is sign of a heart attack. • Assuming friends think your comment is stupid. • Thinking you'll be fired for making a mistake in your report.
Jumping to conclusions	Expecting that a dreaded outcome is extremely likely	• Expecting that you will fail the exam when unsure of a question. • Predicting that your mind will go blank during the speech. • Predicting that you will be extremely anxious if you make the trip.
Tunnel vision	Focusing only on possible threat-relevant information while ignoring evidence of safety	• Noticing that a person looks bored while you are speaking in a meeting. • Focusing exclusively on anxiety symptoms while in the grocery store. • Worrying about a medical test and only thinking it could be positive for cancer.
Nearsightedness	Tendency to assume that threat is imminent	• Socially anxious person thinking every morning she prepares for work that today she could say something embarrassing. • Worry-prone individual being convinced he will be fired any day. • Person with fear of vomiting being concerned she is about to become sick to her stomach because she has an "unsettled feeling."
Emotional reasoning	Assuming that the more intense the anxiety, the greater the actual threat	• "Flying must be dangerous because I feel so anxious when I fly." • Person with panic assuming the likelihood of "losing control" is greater when feeling intense anxiety. • Worry-prone individual being even more convinced something bad will happen because she feels anxious.
All-or-nothing thinking	Viewing threat and safety in rigid, absolute terms as either present or absent	• Person with panic disorder always thinking of having a full-blown panic attack if she feels any anxiety. • Person with social anxiety being convinced his work colleagues will think he is incompetent if he speaks up. • A worrier thinking she will never find a job after being laid off from work.

Note. Reprinted with permission from *Cognitive Therapy of Anxiety Disorders* by David A. Clark and Aaron T. Beck (p. 169). Copyright 2010 by The Guilford Press.

thought "Am I having a heart attack?" Through a series of cognitive errors, Pierre could only think about a possible heart attack and not all the other possible reasons for chest pain, such as that he had just finished his exercise routine or that he'd been drinking too much coffee, or the reasons a heart attack was unlikely, such as that he was young and had no risk factors for heart disease or that he had just had a medical checkup and all was well.

"I Can't Stand This Feeling"

If you've had repeated experiences with intense anxiety over many months, even years, it's understandable that you'd feel frustrated and upset with being anxious. Our patients with anxiety disorders typically exclaim "I just hate this feeling. I would do anything to get rid of it. If only I could feel normal again." Over time people develop certain ideas or beliefs about the experience of anxiety. They tend to catastrophize about being anxious, developing an *intolerance of anxiety* itself. The very experience of anxiety becomes a threat or danger that the person tries to avoid at all costs. The following are some typical beliefs that represent an intolerance for anxiety:

- "I can't stand feeling anxious."
- "If I don't control the anxiety, it will lead to something far worse (cause a heart attack, loss of sanity, loss of complete control, etc.)."
- "Anxiety will continue until I stop it."
- "Anxiety is worse than physical pain, disappointment, or loss."
- "Persistent anxiety can harm your health."
- "Anxiety is a sign that you are losing control."
- "It's important to remain calm and not get so physically keyed up and agitated."

Numerous studies have found that people with anxiety disorders also develop *anxiety sensitivity,* which is fear specifically of the physical sensations of anxiety. When you repeatedly experience anxiety, you may develop a fear of the tension, heart palpitations, and breathlessness experienced during anxiety episodes, believing these symptoms might have serious negative consequences.[19,20] Many people come to dread the physiological arousal of anxiety and so respond quickly to avoid it at all costs.

Another important set of beliefs about anxiety is called *intolerance of uncertainty.* This refers to a tendency to react negatively to unpredictable or uncontrollable situations and events.[21] Most people with intense anxiety prefer the routine and familiar and don't like surprises. The problem is that most of the things that bother them are uncertain because they are in the future. Anxiety over one's health is a common example. We can't be certain we won't get ill, but anxiety disorders can make people intolerant of this uncertainty; they want to know, to be sure, they won't get cancer, have a heart attack, and so on. Ken, for example, had a persistent and excessive fear of cancer. Despite having had numerous medical tests and having been told his health was excellent, he continued to check medical sites on the Internet whenever he experienced an unexplained physical symptom, and he read everything available about early detection of cancer. Ken wanted to know for certain whether he might get cancer. His anxiety was driven by his intolerance of uncertainty and his belief that it was important to reduce uncertainty to an absolute minimum.

A final set of beliefs related to anxiety is *discomfort with novelty, the unfamiliar.* People with frequent anxiety often hate new, unexpected, or unfamiliar situations. Novelty is viewed as threatening. They may believe their anxiety is worse in unfamiliar situations; that they can't cope with novelty. They may seek to stay with the familiar because they believe it is more predictable and controllable. Being in unpredictable and uncontrollable situations is especially difficult for the anxious person. John had social phobia. He often experienced intense anxiety during his encounters with others at work. However, he felt less anxious around people he knew or in highly familiar, routine social situations. Unfamiliar interpersonal situations involving people he didn't know were particularly difficult and anxiety provoking. Consequently, John tried to anticipate whether a situation would be familiar. He would avoid any novel social situations where he might unexpectedly become the focus of other people's attention. These attempts to avoid novel or unfamiliar social situations caused a lot of problems in John's life. It reduced his feelings of anxiety, but at great cost. He continually worried about being confronted unexpectedly with a new social situation, and he frequently avoided important meetings at work for fear that he might be called on to give an opinion. He had actually been passed over for promotion because of his inability to deal with the many unexpected social interactions that occurred at work.

Intolerance Perpetuates Anxiety

Think about it: If you believe that anxiety itself is intolerable, if you come to fear certain physical symptoms of anxiety, or if you believe it's important to be as certain about the future as possible and avoid new or unfamiliar situations, then you're likely to do everything in your power to escape or avoid anxious experiences. You may find yourself on a quest to be anxiety free. But what if the intolerance for anxiety makes you more sensitive to anxiety? Your increased sensitivity to anxiety would become an important contributor to its persistence.

> Cognitive therapy focuses on reducing "anxiety about anxiety" by encouraging greater tolerance for and acceptance of anxiety, its physical symptoms, uncertainty, and the unfamiliar.

Worksheet 3.3 is a Beliefs about Anxiety

scale. Check the box that indicates how strongly you believe each statement about anxiety. Make a note of the belief statements that seem particularly relevant for you. If you're in therapy, you should discuss these with your therapist. You'll come back to this completed worksheet in Chapter 5.

On the Run

The urge to **escape** what you think is causing your anxiety and then to **avoid** any further contact with it is a natural reaction to feeling anxious. Escape and avoidance are the two strategies most commonly used to control anxiety. They are an automatic defensive response to fear and anxiety, and on the surface they seem remarkably effective in stopping anxiety dead in its tracks. Think back to the number of times you felt anxious and left the situation immediately. You are at a party, in a crowded grocery store, at a meeting, driving an unfamiliar route, and you begin to feel intense anxiety. What happens if you immediately leave the situation? More than likely your anxiety subsides almost immediately. Psychologists call this the *fight-or-flight response*. We see it in all animals as well as humans when they are afraid. The natural response is to run or stand your ground and fight. One of our clients, Louise, was afraid of crossing bridges because of a fear of open spaces. For years she had avoided crossing most bridges in her city, which greatly restricted her ability to travel around her community. We met near one of the bridges that Louise avoided with the goal of gradually and systematically approaching the bridge on foot (called *exposure,* described in detail in Chapter 7). As we got within 25 feet of the bridge, I could see that Louise was becoming panicky. Her breathing became shallow, her whole body stiffened, and she stopped dead in her tracks, fear written all over her face. I asked her to describe what she was feeling. She said, "I feel like I can't breathe. My legs have gone weak, and I'm terrified. It's taking everything in my power not to run!"

Running (escape) appears to be the safest option when we're overtaken by anxiety. We quickly learn what objects, situations, or circumstances trigger our anxiety and then avoid future contact with these triggers as much as possible. But the fact that escape and avoidance are natural responses doesn't make them the best anxiety reduction strategies. In fact, clinical researchers and mental health professionals have long known that escape and avoidance are significant contributors to the long-term persistence of anxiety. There are three major problems with escape and avoidance:

1. They prevent anxiety from declining naturally.
2. They prevent you from learning that the dangerous thinking causing the anxiety is false.
3. They come at a great personal cost by limiting what you can do, where you can go, whom you can be with. When you rely on avoidance, you end up believing you are weak, dependent, or inadequate—that you "no longer have a life."

Beliefs about Anxiety

Instructions: Using the 5-point scale at the top of the table, check off your level of agreement with each statement about your anxiety. Try to base your answer on what you've come to believe about your anxiety, not what you think you should believe.

Belief Statements	Completely Disagree	Disagree	Agree	Strongly Agree	Completely Agree
1. I find it very hard to tolerate the feeling of anxiety.					
2. It is important to control anxiety as much as possible.					
3. I try to keep my anxiety episodes as brief as possible.					
4. I frequently avoid situations to prevent anxiety.					
5. I am concerned about the long-term health effects of persistent anxiety.					
6. My anxiety episodes are more distressing than anything else I've experienced.					
7. It is important that I develop better control over anxious thoughts and feelings.					
8. It is important that I not appear anxious or nervous in front of others.					
9. The physical symptoms of anxiety scare me.					
10. I'm concerned the physical symptoms of anxiety could be related to a serious medical problem.					
11. If I don't get better control over my anxiety and worry, I could have a complete mental breakdown.					
12. I am more vulnerable when I am feeling uncertain.					
13. I can't function very well when I am having doubts and uncertainty.					
14. For me the feeling of doubt and uncertainty is upsetting and anxiety provoking.					
15. I try to deal with my uncertainties as quickly as possible.					
16. It is important to avoid the unfamiliar and unexpected because they make me more anxious.					
17. It is important to anticipate the future as much as possible and be prepared for unforeseen circumstances.					

For many years psychologists focused on avoidance of external objects and situations when treating anxiety. But more recently we've discovered that avoidance of thoughts, feelings, and the physical sensations believed to trigger anxiety episodes also contribute to the persistence of anxiety. Some people try to avoid certain thoughts or images that they find anxiety provoking, such as thoughts of death or dying, of saying something rude or embarrassing to others, of imagining some terrible injury happening to a loved one, or of terrible career loss or failure. Others may avoid strong emotional states like excitement, anger, or frustration, believing they are signs of losing control, which they fear could lead to an anxiety episode. Still others might try to avoid anything that causes an increased heart rate, lightheadedness, dizziness, a queasy stomach, shortness of breath, or sweating, because these sensations are also connected with anxiety. We've heard so many individuals with anxiety disorders say, "I won't drink coffee or alcohol because I don't like how it makes me feel."

The following are examples of situations, thoughts, and physical sensations that people with anxiety disorders often try to avoid. Read through the lists. Do any of the entries seem familiar to you? Do you try to avoid any of them to prevent a resurgence of your anxiety?

Situations, Objects, and Other External Cues Often Avoided

- Driving in unfamiliar places
- Being alone at home
- Enclosed places (e.g., elevators, tunnels)
- Dental visits
- Crowds
- Giving a speech
- Initiating a conversation with unfamiliar people
- Answering the phone
- Participating in a meeting
- Walking in front of a group of people

Thoughts, Images, and Impulses Often Avoided

- Disgusting sexual thoughts such as touching a child inappropriately
- Thoughts of causing harm, injury, or death
- Thoughts of bad or catastrophic events happening to friends or loved ones
- Disgusting images such as mutilated bodies
- Thoughts or images of a past personal trauma
- Thoughts or images of embarrassing yourself in front of others

- Thoughts about disease and contamination
- Thoughts of God's punishment or the end of the world
- Doubts about one's sexual orientation
- Thoughts about one's own death

Physical Sensations Often Avoided

- Heart palpitations
- Shortness of breath
- Feeling lightheaded or dizzy
- Sweating
- Queasy stomach or nausea
- Blurred vision
- Feeling blushed
- Feeling sick
- Vomiting

These lists include only a few examples of the many things people might try to avoid so as not to feel anxious. We find that each individual has her own unique avoidance profile. For some it is mainly social or interpersonal situations, for others it may be anything they think might trigger a panic attack, whereas for others it might be upsetting thoughts or images that spontaneously pop into their mind. Whatever we avoid because of anxiety, it is important to discover your unique avoidance profile because it is an important part of the anxious mind-set. Repeated escape and avoidance tends to confirm beliefs that our danger thoughts represent real threats and that we are too weak and vulnerable to stand up to our fears. So reducing our reliance on escape and avoidance is an important goal in cognitive therapy.

Complete Worksheet 3.4 to discover the subtle, and maybe not so subtle, ways that you avoid situations, thoughts, or physical sensations to prevent further anxiety. If you're having trouble identifying your avoidance responses, come back to the worksheet after reading Chapters 5 and 7, which further cover escape and avoidance. (You'll also use this worksheet in Chapter 5.)

⋛ Troubleshooting Tips ⋚

Sometimes it's easy to identify avoidance, such as the agoraphobic person who refuses to go to the shopping mall for fear of a panic attack. At other times the avoidance can be subtle, such as avoiding physical exercise because you dislike the feeling of being out of

Discovering Your Avoidance Profile

Situations, External Triggers	Thoughts, Images, and Impulses	Physical Sensations
Briefly describe any situations, objects, persons, or other external cues that you regularly avoid because of anxiety. List the avoided situations that cause you the greatest interference in your daily living.	List any thoughts, images, or impulses that you try not to think about because they cause you to feel anxious. List the unwanted thoughts that are most distressing or that you try hardest not to think about.	List any specific body sensations, experiences, or symptoms that are especially frightening for you. Do you try to prevent these sensations from happening? If you start to feel the physical symptom or sensation, do you immediately try to control it or suppress it?

breath. To help you identify subtle avoidance of thoughts, images, or physical sensations, consider all activities and experiences that you try to avoid. Ask yourself, "Why do I hate doing this activity? Are there particular thoughts or physical sensations that I would rather not have, that I am trying to avoid?" You can review the previous list to see if you might be avoiding some of these thoughts and feelings in the situation. If you're being treated for anxiety, your therapist should be able to help you identify "subtle avoidance."

Searching for Safety

When feeling anxious, people often say, "If only I could calm down, relax, or just take things as they come." In other words, when we perceive threat or danger and feel anxious, our desire is to "feel safe." This desire for calm and comfort leads us to engage in safety-seeking behaviors. *Safety seeking* is:

> Cognitive therapy helps people reduce and eventually eliminate unhealthy avoidance patterns so that anxiety can be allowed to decline naturally.

any cognitive or behavioral response intended to prevent or minimize a feared outcome. It is also an attempt to reestablish a feeling of comfort or calm and a sense of being safe. [22,23]

Escape and avoidance are the most common safety-seeking behaviors used to prevent or minimize anxiety, but they're not the only ones. Put a check mark beside the behaviors and thoughts that you use to avoid anxiety or discuss them with your therapist.

Behavioral Safety Seeking

- Leave (escape) when first symptoms of anxiety are noticed
- Carry antianxiety medication
- Carry cell phone to call for help when anxious
- Be accompanied by friend or family member in anxious situations
- Have water or other liquids readily available
- Listen to music when anxious
- Engage in relaxation or controlled breathing when anxious
- Lie down, rest when anxious
- Whistle, sing to yourself
- Tense or hold on to objects when anxious

■ Distract yourself by looking away from whatever evokes fear

■ Seek reassurance from others

Cognitive Safety Seeking

■ Think about something more positive or calming

■ Try to imagine yourself in a safe or peaceful situation

■ Try to reassure yourself that everything will be all right

■ Try to convince yourself you're not really feeling anxious

■ Try to focus on the task at hand, such as work or driving, to avoid attending to the anxiety

■ Pray; seek divine protection

■ Criticize yourself for feeling anxious

What's Wrong with Seeking Safety?

Trying to feel calm and safe seems like a good idea, but there are four drawbacks to safety seeking:

1. It's more difficult to process safety cues than danger or threat cues.
2. The emphasis is on immediate fear reduction, which means you can end up relying on inappropriate safety-seeking strategies.
3. It prevents you from learning your perception of threat or danger is false.
4. It reinforces the unrealistic desire to eliminate all risk.

It may be harder to know whether a situation is safe than to determine whether it holds the potential for danger.[23] For example, if you walk into a social gathering, you may find it quite easy to quickly pick out cues that other people don't accept you—maybe someone frowns at you or glances at you and then immediately continues a conversation with someone else. It is much harder to recognize the cues indicating they accept you; you may not realize that a smile is intended for you or that someone is looking at you to include you in a conversation. Because it's harder to process information that would make you feel comfortable and safe, you might tend to rely on strategies that will quickly reduce your anxiety. If so, you won't learn that the situation is not really threatening and you'll keep trying to minimize perceived risk as quickly as possible. Your safety-seeking efforts will have contributed to a persistence of the anxiety problem.

When Louise tried to approach the river with her therapist, she had a bottle of fruit juice with her, ostensibly to offset dry mouth. But when her anxiety increased,

> Cognitive therapy can help you attain real comfort and security by eliminating ineffective safety-seeking behaviors and improving your ability to truly appreciate the actual safety features of situations that make you feel anxious.

she practically guzzled the juice, indicating that the juice was a safety-seeking response. Then, when she approached the edge of the sidewalk to look down at the river, she held tightly on to the railing that ran along the walkway. Clinging to the railing was another safety-seeking response. Interestingly, she had a very difficult time processing the real safety feature of the situation: that she was standing on a sidewalk 100 feet from the river with a chest-high railing in front of her.

Preparing for the Worst

If you think something bad or terrible is about to happen, it makes sense to want to prepare for the worst. It's only natural to try to problem-solve about how you would deal with catastrophes like having a full-blown panic attack, having your mind go blank in front of an audience, or having your computer hacked because you forgot to shut it down. The attempt to prepare for bad or threatening possibilities when feeling anxious is called worry. *Worry* is:

> *a persistent chain of repetitive, uncontrollable thinking that focuses on uncertain future negative outcomes. It involves repeated mental rehearsal of possible solutions that fail to resolve the sense of uncertainty about an impending threat.*

Worry is a very common feature of anxiety. We worry about having another panic attack; whether our health will fail and we'll get a horrible disease, like cancer, that has not yet been detected; that harm or injury will occur to our children; that people think we are incompetent; that we'll lose our job and be left in financial ruin; and a million other possible events. The list of potential worry concerns truly is endless. Although certain worry themes are common in the anxiety disorders, the specific things that worry us most can be unique to each individual. And worry occurs naturally, automatically in people with anxiety problems. In decades of treating anxious individuals, we have never met an anxious person who had to "work harder at worrying." No one has said, "You know, at first I was a really bad worrier, but with years of practice I can now say that I've mastered the art of excessive worry!!"

So if worry is as natural to the anxious person as breathing, what's the problem? We've learned that worry is a problem in anxiety because:

- It keeps your focus on thoughts of threat and danger.

- It reinforces a sense of personal helplessness because it's difficult to control.

■ It fuels a sense of uncertainty because it's always future oriented, and the future is unknowable.

■ It is an avoidance of the core fear that underlies anxiety problems.

The adverse effects of worry are illustrated by Ron, who was anxious about his health. Ron's fear that he might have cancer or develop a brain tumor compelled him to scan his body constantly for aches, pains, or unusual physical sensations. When he detected a red spot or skin rash, he would fret over the possibility that it might be skin cancer. His worry got him nowhere, because he got stuck on thoughts like these: "What if this is skin cancer?" "How can I be sure it's not skin cancer?" "Maybe it could be precancerous and I'll eventually develop skin cancer, or maybe it's too early to tell whether it's cancer." Although Ron tried to calm his worries by searching through medical websites, asking friends and relatives if they thought the spot was cancer, even scheduling repeated consults with his family physician, he remained anxious about the spot until it disappeared. Ron's worry was a major contributor to his anxiety because it ensured that he remained focused on threat ("This red spot could be cancer"). Also he felt helpless in the face of his inability to shut down the worry, and it kept him locked into the uncertainties of the future (nobody can possibly know what the next day holds!). Interestingly, Ron's worry about the red spot and whether it was cancerous meant that he avoided dealing with his core fear of being diagnosed with cancer and the possibility of death.

If worry is an important factor in your anxiety, Chapter 11 will be especially relevant since it's devoted to worry. Meanwhile, use Worksheet 3.5 to write down what you worry about when feeling anxious. You will use this information if you choose to work through Chapter 11.

> Our cognitive therapy program can teach you how to turn excessive worry into realistic problem solving so that worry does not keep you focused on imagined future threat or danger.

Preparing for Action

To benefit from cognitive therapy, you need to understand how your anxious mind works—why your anxiety persists because of how your brain automatically processes threat and safety information. In this chapter we discussed eight aspects of anxious thinking that contribute to the persistence of anxiety:

■ Automatic catastrophic thinking

■ Helplessness beliefs about anxiety

■ Cognitive errors about threat/danger

■ Heightened sensitivity to feeling anxious

List of My Anxious Worries

Instructions: There may be a number of things that worry you, or your worry may focus on one or two main themes. For the moment, make a preliminary list of your anxious worries.

1. _____

   _____

2. _____

   _____

3. _____

   _____

4. _____

   _____

5. _____

   _____

- Low tolerance for the unfamiliar and for uncertainty
- Reliance on escape and avoidance
- Search for calm and safety
- Excessive worry

You now have an understanding of how these various components of anxiety link together to maintain anxiety—a critical step in overcoming fear and anxiety. You're almost ready to take the first step in your cognitive therapy program, which involves conducting a more specific assessment of the various aspects of your anxious thinking and behavior to create a "map" of how *you* think anxiously. That map will emerge from your work in Chapter 5 and will provide the foundation for a cognitive intervention that you will develop in Chapter 8. First, though, as you would for, let's say, starting a physical fitness program, it's important to prepare: take a look at your assumptions and expectations and figure out how ready you are to commit to a program.

CHAPTER SUMMARY

- Anxiety will decline naturally unless an anxious mind-set is activated that ensures its repeated occurrence and persistence.

- Automatic thoughts and images that exaggerate (i.e., overestimate) the likelihood and severity of threats or dangers in ordinary everyday situations (i.e., catastrophizing or dangerous thinking) are the core fear that underlies persistent anxiety.

- Anxious individuals tend to think of themselves as weak, helpless, and vulnerable, so they underestimate their ability to cope with their fearful concerns.

- When anxious, people tend to make a number of thinking errors, so they remain selectively focused on threat and danger.

- Over time, anxious people develop an intolerance for anxiety, its physical symptoms, and a sense of uncertainty so they become "anxious about being anxious."

- Anxious people are often intolerant of uncertainty and feel highly uncomfortable in novel or unfamiliar situations, which can lead to a life that feels like "death by boredom."

- Escape and avoidance are the most common unhelpful coping strategies associated with persistent anxiety.

- Anxious individuals often rely on inappropriate safety-seeking strategies to obtain immediate relief from anxiety and reestablish a sense of comfort and security.

- Worry is a common characteristic of persistent anxiety that contributes to a preoccupation with threat and danger.

4

Getting Started

When you hear about the importance of being fit, you undoubtedly think of physical fitness. Every day we're bombarded with messages emphasizing the importance of staying active and healthy. But what about **mental fitness**? A command surgeon in the U.S. Army has described mental fitness as "having the psychological strength, ability, and freedom to efficiently and successfully manage the stresses, problems, adversities, painful emotions, and frustrations in daily living."[24] Sounds every bit as desirable as physical fitness, doesn't it?

Generally, we know what it takes to achieve physical fitness: a regular training program that keeps our bodies strong, agile, and resilient. The same is true for the mind. We can become psychologically and emotionally stronger by engaging in a daily training program in a similar fashion to regular physical exercise. We can reduce the damaging impact of anxiety on our lives just as we can counteract the modern sedentary lifestyle. That's what cognitive therapy and this workbook are all about.

As anyone who's embarked on a physical fitness program knows, however, recognizing that regular exercise and a balanced diet are important is the easy part. Actually putting this principle into practice—well, that's a far different story. Initial enthusiasm wanes, schedules collapse, resolve crumbles, excuses start to sound more and more reasonable. Even the most die-hard fitness enthusiasts find regular exercise tough. Fortunately, those who make some effort to stick with it find that the benefits—both long- and short-term—become so deeply ingrained that they miss exercising when they let their regimen lapse. We believe you'll discover the same when you devote your energy to the work in this book. That's why this chapter is important: arming yourself with the mental tools you need to keep working at reducing your anxiety will give you a chance to recognize the benefits and make the cognitive approach work for you.

Different Starting Points

Each of us may start at different points on the pathway to mental fitness and wholeness. Because of previous life adversities, childhood difficulties, family history, biological predispositions, and other factors, some people may have to work harder at mental fitness than others. But everyone can improve his or her mental fitness. Have you ever made a commitment to yourself to improve your emotional health? Maybe you've tried some kind of therapy but have not been satisfied with the results or enjoyed lasting improvements. If so, be assured that this workbook has been designed to help you make long-term changes, just as cognitive therapy has been shown to have long-term beneficial effects on anxiety. Are you ready to make some changes, to improve yourself psychologically so you are better able to meet the challenges and adversities of daily living?

> As with physical fitness, it takes committed action to maintain mental and emotional fitness. Cognitive therapy is a mental fitness training program that will build your psychological strength so you can face the stresses, fears, and anxieties of daily living.

What Are Mental Self-Help Exercises?

Research studies have shown that individuals who engage in **homework assignments** between cognitive therapy sessions experience greater improvements in anxiety or depression than individuals who don't.[25,26] And obviously homework is critical to a self-help workbook.

In this workbook, homework or self-help **exercises** are defined as:

any specific, clearly defined, structured activity that is carried out in a person's home, work, or community to observe, evaluate, or modify the faulty cognitions and maladaptive behaviors that characterize anxiety.

For example, Darrell avoids public places because he believes being there causes his panic attacks. His mental self-help exercises need to focus on demonstrating to him that it is not the places that trigger anxiety but his tendency to misinterpret his increased heart rate as a sign of a possible heart attack. Jessica constantly worried about almost every aspect of her life—the health of her daughters, the viability of her marriage, the future of her aging mother, and so forth. Her exercises needed to test her beliefs that worrying was preparing her for the worst. Deborah feels extremely anxious in anticipation of all social situations, because she's convinced she is the only person who feels this level of anxiety and that embarrassing herself is inevitable. Her exercises would be focused on showing her not only that many people feel some level of social anxiety but also that they can perform well even while anxious.

Maybe you're thinking that this sounds good but is a lot easier said than done. You may bring to this book (or to therapy) a lot of preconceived notions about the effectiveness of self-help exercises and about cognitive therapy techniques in general. You'll see for yourself if you do the exercises that cognitive therapy tools and techniques have been crafted meticulously to anticipate stumbling blocks and help you chip away at the negative effects of anxiety in your life. But if you have doubts that could keep you from diving in, now is the time to clear away any preconceived notions that are standing in your way. We've found that when people have trouble completing the homework, either as self-help or with a therapist's guidance, the problem often lies in preconceived notions about this work. You might feel eager to tackle your anxiety and believe you're entering this program with an open mind, but little doubts and questions often lurk in the back of people's minds, ready to pop up and sabotage their efforts when they least expect it. Exposing these hobgoblins to the light of day and addressing them now will help you get the most out of the work you do in this book and/or in therapy.

> You will get more from treatment or self-help if you fill out the worksheets and questionnaires. In fact, one of the most common reasons for lack of progress is failure to do cognitive therapy homework exercises.

If you want to see an improvement in your anxiety, be prepared to do your homework!

What Are Your Beliefs about Cognitive Therapy Exercises?

Are you fully aware of the beliefs you hold about the self-help or homework exercises involved with cognitive therapy? Take a few minutes and rate yourself on the belief statements in Worksheet 4.1.

How did you do? We don't have data that will tell you reliably what ratings indicate being ready for cognitive therapy. But you can use the checklist more informally by looking over the belief statements for which you checked off "agree" or "strongly agree." All of these statements reflect ideas that might interfere with your ability to commit to this program. Here are a few ideas for how you can use the information from the worksheet to overcome your reluctance to engage in self-improvement of anxiety.

- **Write** down the "agree" and "strongly agree" items on a piece of paper.
- **Question** the accuracy of these beliefs. What are the consequences for you of holding these beliefs? Are there any errors or distortions in your thinking (see Table 3.2)?
- **Substitute** the term "physically fit or unfit" for "anxiety" in your belief state-

Identifying Your Beliefs about Self-Help Assignments

Instructions: Please read each statement and circle the number that best corresponds with how much you agree or disagree with each belief about self-help exercises.

Belief Statement	Strongly Disagree	Disagree	Agree	Strongly Agree
1. Doing these assignments will make my anxiety worse.	1	2	3	4
2. There is no point in trying; nothing can help me.	1	2	3	4
3. I should not have to practice skills to overcome my anxiety.	1	2	3	4
4. I am too anxious to do homework tasks right now.	1	2	3	4
5. My anxiety has been pretty good; I don't want to risk making things worse by doing self-help exercises.	1	2	3	4
6. I don't believe these exercises are an effective approach for reducing anxiety.	1	2	3	4
7. I am a procrastinator; I've always had trouble motivating myself to do extra work.	1	2	3	4
8. I'm not getting any better, so why bother doing these exercises?	1	2	3	4
9. I'm too tired or stressed to do self-help exercises.	1	2	3	4
10. These tasks are trivial; I don't see how this will help me beat anxiety.	1	2	3	4
11. I'm too busy and don't have time for daily mental self-help exercises.	1	2	3	4

(cont.)

Belief Statement	Strongly Disagree	Disagree	Agree	Strongly Agree
12. Anxiety is a medical condition; I shouldn't have to go to all this effort to get rid of it.	1	2	3	4
13. Other people overcome anxiety without putting this much work into it.	1	2	3	4
14. There is a deep-seated root to my anxiety that needs to be discovered; I don't see how these exercises can be effective.	1	2	3	4
15. What if I don't do these exercises correctly and they make my anxiety worse?	1	2	3	4
16. I hate writing things down; I've never been a person to keep records.	1	2	3	4
17. I lack the motivation and discipline to do this kind of therapy.	1	2	3	4
18. This is too hard; there must be an easier way to overcome anxiety.	1	2	3	4
19. Doing even a little homework is better than doing nothing at all.	1	2	3	4
20. Even if I don't do the self-help exercises, going to therapy sessions or reading about anxiety should be somewhat helpful.	1	2	3	4
21. I've always hated doing homework, even as a child.	1	2	3	4
22. I don't like following rigid programs; I prefer to do things my own way.	1	2	3	4
23. I can overcome my anxiety without doing these homework assignments.	1	2	3	4
24. I've made progress on my anxiety in the past without doing self-help exercises; therefore I shouldn't need to do them now.	1	2	3	4
25. These exercises are too demanding; I just don't see how they are going to help me overcome anxiety.	1	2	3	4

ment (e.g., "I can overcome my *physical unfitness* without doing these home-work assignments"). Would you believe this statement if it referred to getting physically fit? If it is untrue for physical fitness, how can it be true for mental fitness? You could discuss with friends how they have overcome some of these beliefs in terms of a physical fitness program.

▪ **Take action** by doing something small that might test out or correct the belief (e.g., if you believe you lack the discipline to do self-help assignments [Item 17], you could start by engaging in a brief, limited self-help exercise that takes only a few minutes each day).

ꗥ Troubleshooting Tips ꗦ

If you still have some doubts about your readiness to do the exercises in this workbook, and you are in therapy, you should discuss these doubts with your therapist, which could also be a roadblock to your therapy progress. If you are reading the workbook on your own, talk to others who overcame anxiety through therapy. What role did exercise play in their recovery? Also, we are not asking you to do all the exercises all the time. Instead we are asking you to **set aside just 20–30 minutes on most days and focus on one exercise at a time.** Do you recall the old Chinese saying "Every journey begins with the first step"? That's our outlook in cognitive therapy. You have already taken the first step by getting this far in the workbook. Are you ready to continue the journey toward recovery?

What Have You Heard about Cognitive Therapy?

You probably wouldn't have gotten this far in the book if you had serious doubts about the cognitive therapy approach to anxiety. But if you've been exposed to the following misconceptions about cognitive therapy, they could weaken your confidence or motivation while you're working your way through this book. Let's put them to rest once and for all:

Myth: Cognitive therapy is overly intellectual and does not deal with feelings.

Fact: *It is true that cognitive therapy focuses a lot on how we think and behave. But the thoughts and beliefs important in cognitive therapy are emotional— they deal with our emotions and not our intellect. Cognitive therapy is all about changing emotions, and in this workbook we continually ask people to observe, record, and understand "how they feel."*

Myth: Only well-educated or highly intelligent people can benefit from cognitive therapy.

Fact: *The ability to observe your thinking, evaluate it, and consider alternative ways of thinking is more important to the success of cognitive therapy than how far you went in school or your IQ.*

Myth: Because it's very rigid, cognitive therapy can't take into account the unique needs and circumstances of individuals.

Fact: *Cognitive therapy is always applied to the unique features of a person's anxious experience, as you will find in the next chapter when you work on your anxiety profile.*

Myth: Cognitive therapy is very superficial, dealing only with symptoms and not addressing the root cause of anxiety.

Fact: *As you'll recall from Chapter 3, cognitive therapy considers automatic thoughts and beliefs about threat and helplessness basic elements of anxiety. By addressing these cognitive "root causes," cognitive therapy has often shown more enduring benefits for reducing anxiety than medication.*

Myth: You can't benefit from cognitive therapy if you're taking medication for anxiety.

Fact: *Research studies and our own clinical experience have shown that people on medication for anxiety can benefit significantly from cognitive therapy.*

Myth: You have to be well organized and disciplined to benefit from cognitive therapy.

Fact: *There is no research evidence that a well-organized and disciplined personality type benefits more from cognitive therapy than anyone else.*

Myth: Cognitive therapy completely ignores the influence of one's past.

Fact: *Cognitive therapy does focus on the present, but past difficult experiences and childhood adversities may be considered when they have an important influence on individuals' present emotional functioning.*

Myth: Cognitive therapy is effective only with mild or moderate anxiety.

Fact: *Research outcome studies that have formally evaluated cognitive therapy have shown that individuals with severe anxiety symptoms and disorders can achieve significant symptom improvement.*

Myth: Cognitive therapy is only "talk therapy" in which people "talk themselves out of being anxious."

Fact: *Behavior change is a very important part of cognitive therapy. Although changing one's thinking about anxiety is critical, it is just as important that people also change their behavior and act differently in response to their anxiety.*

Myth: Cognitive therapy emphasizes the "power of positive thinking" to trick people into being less anxious.

Fact: *Cognitive therapy emphasizes the importance of "realistic thinking" and not "positive thinking." It reduces anxiety by teaching people to replace unrealistic, exaggerated thinking with more accurate, realistic evaluations of threat in ordinary daily activities.*

Myth: Cognitive treatment for anxiety is slow and can take many weeks before real benefits are seen.

Fact: *Many of the significant effects of cognitive therapy are seen in the first few sessions. You can expect to see some improvement within the first 4 to 6 weeks of cognitive therapy.*

Myth: It is rare to see sudden anxiety reductions in cognitive therapy.

Fact: *People in formal cognitive therapy can experience a sudden reduction in anxiety from one week to the next. It is unknown whether these sudden changes occur when using cognitive therapy self-help.*

⋛ Troubleshooting Tips ⋚

If you hit a point in this workbook where you feel stalled or unmotivated, come back to this list and see whether you still subscribe to any of these myths. If so, remind yourself of the facts. Or it may be that you believe one of these "myths" about cognitive therapy and it's preventing you from committing to this workbook program. If this is the case, consider whether you can suspend judgment about the cognitive therapy approach until you've given it a try. You could select some aspect of your anxiety experiences and use one or two exercises in Chapters 6 or 7 over a 2- to 3-week period. Observe what effect it has had on your anxiety. Is it worth continuing? The best evidence for the approach will be your own experience. If you're working with a cognitive therapist, discuss your concerns with your therapist. After observing the effects of these exercises, you may be ready to implement the full cognitive therapy program you will set up in Chapter 8.

Maximizing Your Success

Besides shedding myths and other nonproductive preconceived notions about doing the work in this book, there are several measures you can adopt to make your efforts as fruitful as they can be.

Effective Self-Help Exercises

First, look at the construction of any self-help exercise you're about to do to make sure it contains the elements that contribute to success. Not all self-help exercises are created equal. A poorly constructed exercise can be ineffective at best, and downright harmful at worst.

For many years Earl, age 44, suffered from intense anxiety caused by upsetting, intrusive thoughts of harm or injury to loved ones. For example, he had thoughts of a friend being in a car accident and then became anxious that this might really happen, or he would think of a family member having a serious illness and then worry that he or she might actually become seriously sick. Earl experienced these terrible thoughts many times throughout the day and tried to distract himself from the thoughts or reassure himself that everything would be all right.

To overcome the anxiety caused by these worrisome thoughts, it was important for Earl to engage in exercises that exposed him to situations that triggered the worry, practice correcting his automatic thoughts of danger (e.g., "If I have this worry about harm, maybe something bad will happen to people"), and prevent efforts to control the worry. Earl, however, was never very keen on doing these homework tasks. He was quite happy to attend therapy sessions and talk about his anxiety, but he had great difficulty finding the time to apply the therapy. Earl tried to do some of the things his cognitive therapist recommended, but they never worked for him. He was afraid the exercises would make him feel more anxious. He was impatient with the pace of therapy and felt like the exercises were trivial and unimportant. He refused to keep a written account of the exercises and would do them only once or twice a week for a few minutes. He said he was too busy and didn't have enough time. When he did an exercise, he would stop it as soon as he felt a little anxious. In the end, the whole process was frustrating and unproductive for Earl. Despite faithfully attending his therapy sessions, Earl was unable to overcome his anxious, worrisome thoughts.

Keys to an Effective Self-Help Exercise

What went wrong? Missing from Earl's efforts were a number of ingredients that are critical to an effective self-help exercise:

1. **Clear rationale**   The exercise must address an important aspect of persistent anxiety and must contribute to your goal of anxiety reduction.

2. **Cost–benefits review**   Before starting a self-help exercise, you should be clear about the costs and benefits associated with investing in the exercise.

3. **Precise description**   The exercise should be clearly specified so you know exactly what to do, when, and for how long. In addition, state the outcome or goal you would like to achieve with the exercise.

4. **Graduated steps**   Each exercise should be a component of a systematic exercise program in which you start with something at a lower anxiety level and work up to situations or tasks that involve intense anxiety.

5. **Record keeping**   A brief written description of your behavior, thinking, and anxiety level should be recorded each time you engage in a self-help exercise. Good record keeping is an essential part of a systematic, effective self-help mental exercise program.

6. **Practice, practice, practice!**   Do each exercise repeatedly and frequently, possibly even daily, before moving on to the next level. Just like physical exercise, most treatments for anxiety fail because people don't spend enough time doing self-help exercises.

7. **Evaluate and problem-solve**   After completing an exercise session, evaluate your success at doing the exercise and its effect on your anxiety. Did you achieve your stated goal? If you didn't, what barriers did you encounter? How can you improve on the exercise the next time you do it?

Earl wasn't sure of the benefits he stood to gain from doing the exercises assigned by his therapist, he didn't stick with the tasks and work his way up gradually, he refused to keep a written record of his exercise experiences, he didn't practice regularly, and he never tried to determine what had gone wrong and how he might rectify the problems.

Belinda, age 32, who wanted to address intense social anxiety, took advantage of all the arrows in the cognitive therapy quiver. Belinda felt conspicuous around others and believed that people could see she was anxious and therefore conclude that she must have an emotional problem. Her self-help exercises exposed her to increasingly more intense anxiety-provoking social situations. She practiced these exercises on a daily basis and recorded her progress in structured diaries and rating forms. If she had trouble with a particular exercise, she wrote it down on her evaluation form and then problem-solved the issues. She also used the exercises as an opportunity to practice correcting her exaggerated thoughts of fear and danger and to refine her coping responses to anxiety. After several weeks of daily structured exercise, Belinda found she was much less anxious in a variety of common social situations, and she felt much more confident in her social skills.

The people you met at the beginning of this chapter—Darrell, Jessica, and Deborah—also used exercises that helped them.

Darrell's exercises involved going into the supermarket in the morning when only a few people were shopping. He would stay close to the front of the store, near the exit, and monitor his anxiety level, note any physical symptoms, and identify any anxious thoughts or interpretations of the symptoms. He then generated alternative, less frightening interpretations of his physical symptoms. Darrell did not leave the store until his anxiety level had declined to 50% of its highest level when he entered the store. Also Darrell practiced going to the store every day until he gained mental fitness in that situation—that is, he could enter the front of the store without feeling intense anxiety. Once this situation was conquered, he proceeded to a new anxiety situation, such as shopping for prolonged periods throughout the store.

In therapy, Jessica learned the difference between productive and unproductive worry (if you're not in therapy, you can learn a lot about this distinction in Chapter 11). She was given a sheet that listed the characteristics of both types of worry. Over the next week, Jessica's therapist asked her to record several worry episodes each day and to indicate whether the worry met the criteria of productive or unproductive worry. She was amazed to learn that two-thirds of her worry was unproductive and had little to do with preparing her for future negative events. Her therapist then used this information to evaluate some of her faulty beliefs about worry and to structure various strategies she could use in response to unproductive worry. For Jessica, mental fitness involved actively monitoring her worry and learning to view it from this new perspective.

As noted earlier, one of Deborah's core beliefs was that she is the only person who gets anxious and that anxiety always leads to embarrassment. To test out this belief, Deborah's therapist asked her to observe and rate other people's anxiety level at the next meeting. She was to write down any outward signs of anxiety she observed in others and to rate their probable level of anxiety on a 0 to 100 scale. She was also asked to record how well they performed at the meeting in spite of their anxiety. This self-help exercise played a critical role in Deborah's learning that anxiety is common and does not always lead to a disastrous outcome; that a person can perform quite well even when anxious. By changing some old attitudes about anxiety, Deborah was gaining strength to actually try expressing her opinion despite feeling very anxious.

These three people gained improvement through self-help exercises by working on their anxieties *one at a time,* by addressing each anxiety *gradually,* and by *sticking with the exercise even though their anxiety rose initially* when they were exposed to their fear. It's just like physical fitness: you begin at a level that is only slightly challenging, you build strength gradually, and you subscribe to the "no pain, no gain" principle if you really want to get stronger. And just as with physical fitness, there are some "rules" to keep in mind that will enhance your chances of improvement:

Rules for Success

1. **Make time for yourself.** If you ever start questioning whether you can spare the time to do the cognitive therapy exercises in this book, stop and consider how much time you waste now because of anxiety. Have you ever sat down and figured out how much time you spend each day worrying, feeling tired because of insomnia, being stressed out, or being unproductive because of avoidance? Now compare this to how much time is needed to do the exercises. Would an investment in anxiety reduction now cause a net loss or gain in time and productivity in the coming months?

2. **Start low and work up.** You've heard the saying "Rome wasn't built in a day." This certainly applies to cognitive therapy for anxiety. If you are very sensitive to, even intolerant of, anxiety (see Chapter 3), it's important not to overwhelm yourself by trying to do too much. It's much better to start with something that causes only mild or moderate anxiety and then gradually work up to more intense anxiety situations.

3. **Pace yourself.** If you've ever done a road race, you'll know that keeping a good steady pace is the key to finishing the race. The same is true for your cognitive therapy program. It's better to do a little each day and every day than to do nothing for a few days and then do something for a couple of hours on the weekend. Read a little of the workbook each day and make sure you spend at least a little time on the exercises.

4. **Keep written records.** There is no substitute for recording your experiences. Written records are important because they help break the automatic responses that make up anxiety episodes. Sorry—no shortcuts; you need to write out your homework tasks.

5. **Catch the thoughts.** When doing cognitive therapy exercises, focus on how you are thinking. If you feel anxious, write down thoughts of exaggerated threat and danger (i.e., catastrophic thinking). Are there errors or distortions in your thinking?

Are you convinced you're helpless or can't stand the anxiety? Are you thinking about escape or relying on a false sense of safety? Becoming more aware of your anxious thinking and learning to correct it (see Chapter 6) is an important strategy for reducing anxiety.

6. Be patient and don't give up. When anxiety is building and the anxious mind takes over, one's instinct is to run! Although this is entirely understandable, it's important to stick with the exercise. Don't leave the situation or give up. Break time into small units and focus on reaching the next goal (e.g., "I'll stay for 10 more minutes, and once that is reached, I'll stay for another 10 minutes, and so on"). This is how runners finish a race when they are tired, aching, and want to give up.

7. Celebrate success and problem-solve barriers. Many people who begin a cognitive therapy program see improvements in their anxiety right away. It is important to recognize your achievements and celebrate the progress you've made in overcoming anxiety. After all, you're the one who made the changes, and so you need to encourage yourself. At the same time, expect setbacks and disappointments. Instead of giving up, take a close look at why the assignment did not go well. Take a problem-oriented approach and see what changes you can make to break through the failed attempt.

As with any fitness program, daily practice in applying cognitive and behavioral strategies to your anxiety experiences will determine the effectiveness of the treatment. Taking a realistic, consistent, and determined approach to the exercises will enhance the anxiety-reducing effects of cognitive therapy.

8. Don't fight anxiety; let it flow. Anxiety is like being entangled in a net; the more you fight it, the worse the entanglement. Take note of whether you are trying to control your anxiety when doing the self-help exercises. Fighting for control will make your anxiety worse. Instead, focus on accepting your anxious state and allowing the anxiety to decline naturally (see Chapter 2 for review).

Completing the Worksheets

We can't emphasize enough the importance of written records in changing the beliefs that fuel anxiety. You'll be filling out two kinds of worksheets in this book: (1) rating scales and diaries for recording your anxiety triggers, your reactions to them, and other parts of your experience with anxiety; and (2) forms for planning, carrying out, and recording your efforts to tackle specific anxiety problems. You've already completed some of the first kind in earlier chapters, and you're going to fill out more of these in Chapter 5. Once you start working on particular anxiety triggers using cognitive therapy methods you've chosen from Chapters 6 and 7, you'll be using the second kind of worksheet—but at the same time, you'll continue rating your anxiety as a way to track your progress, identify obstacles, and revise your game plan. Here are some tips for making the most of both kinds of worksheets.

■ Always fill out the worksheets on your own so that you capture your perspective on your anxiety.

■ Follow the instructions provided on the worksheet and try to answer any specific questions that appear on the worksheet.

■ Don't spend a lot of time worrying about whether your entries on the worksheets are entirely precise or accurate. You'll get better at doing this type of work as time progresses.

■ Avoid being a "perfectionist." Your worksheets don't have to be perfect, but always consider them a "work in progress"—an opportunity to learn.

■ Be sure to carry with you the worksheets you are supposed to fill out during or right after an anxiety episode.

■ Try to complete the worksheets as close to an anxiety experience as possible. If you wait until hours or days later, you'll forget a lot of valuable information about your experience.

■ Resist the temptation to go back and change your entries to worksheets already completed. Your first, immediate response on a worksheet is probably the best.

⇗ Troubleshooting Tips ⇙

Did you have difficulty completing the worksheets in the last chapter? If so, review your entries on the worksheets after you've read this chapter. Identify where you may have gone wrong and make corrections in how you approach the self-help exercises. For example, were you being a perfectionist? Or were you waiting too long after an anxiety episode to complete the worksheet? These are things that you can change as you work through the exercises in the coming chapters. If you are in therapy, discuss your practical problems with the homework exercises with your therapist.

CHAPTER SUMMARY

■ Mental fitness is needed to meet the stresses, anxieties, and fears of contemporary life.

■ Despite our different temperaments and life experiences, improvement in mental and emotional health does not occur accidentally. It requires commitment to change and the adoption of an effective training program.

■ The cognitive therapy described in this workbook is a mental fitness training program for reduction of fear and anxiety.

■ Completing self-help exercises is a critical component of cognitive therapy for anxiety. For treatment to be successful, you must put into practice the knowledge and skills learned from the workbook. It's a simple fact: Consistent completion of worksheet exercises equals greater improvement in anxiety.

■ An effective self-help exercise should have a solid rationale, a precise description, be systematic and gradual, involve a written component and evaluation, and encourage repeated daily practice.

■ Determine whether you hold any negative beliefs or expectations that undermine your motivation to engage in self-help assignments (see Worksheet 4.1). Evaluate the negative consequences of holding on to these beliefs and consider a more balanced and realistic perspective that would encourage better engagement in the cognitive therapy exercises.

■ Make room in your day to work on your anxiety. Schedule a specific time and location for completing self-help assignments.

■ Adopt a balanced, realistic understanding and expectation for your anxiety-reduction training program. Make note and modify any beliefs about cognitive therapy that might interfere in your acceptance of this workbook program.

Maximize the workbook's effectiveness by including the workbook exercises into your daily living. Use the exercises to practice your skill in catching anxious thinking and to refine your coping skills during anxious episodes. Above all, let anxiety subside naturally and continue to PRACTICE, PRACTICE, PRACTICE the workbook cognitive and behavioral skills in real-life anxious situations.

5

Developing Your Anxiety Profile

A 36-year-old mother, we'll call her Beth, enters my office and sits in the chair across from my desk. She sits quietly, with downcast eyes, waiting for me to make a comment. It is obvious that she's nervous and that this is the first time she has seen a therapist. After the usual introductions I ask Beth why she made the appointment. As she begins to tell me her story, I notice that her body is tense, her voice is strained, and she shifts frequently in her seat. This whole process is clearly anxiety provoking for her.

Beth, it turns out, has panic attacks. Her surges of anxiety are so great that she has been missing a lot of work. Recently she was put on notice for excessive absenteeism and is in danger of losing her job. The panic attacks and daily anxiety and worry were debilitating in many other ways as well. Beth was becoming "people phobic." Because her anxiety was much worse in social situations, she started avoiding crowds, then social gatherings, next smaller events like dinner invitations and visiting new friends, and now she won't interact with her closest friends or family members. She won't even return their phone calls or text messages. Except for work, Beth has become practically housebound, her home becoming her only "safe haven" from anxiety. Her husband is exasperated because she won't go anywhere or have contact with anyone. Anxiety is ruining Beth's life, and her job and marriage could be next!

In our first sessions Beth revealed a number of other factors that had weakened her ability to deal with her anxiety. In the last two years she had moved up north so her husband could take a new position with his company. She did not like her new community and missed her old friends. She was now a few hundred miles from her family, whom she rarely saw because anxiety made it difficult for her to travel. Her job at a call center was a definite case of underemployment, but it was all she could get. To make matters worse, her 10-year-old son was having difficulty at his new school, and her 8-year-old daughter longed for her old friends. Everyone in the family is feeling miserable and upset—everyone, that is, except Beth's husband, whose promotion has required more travel. Beth is feeling lonely, discouraged, and scared for her future and that of her family.

As with Beth's, anxiety is complicated, and everyone's story, circumstances, and experiences are unique. If you're working with a therapist, she or he must spend time asking questions, probing, summarizing, and interpreting interview and question-naire responses to get a thorough understanding of the complexities of the person's anxiety. Cognitive therapists assess anxiety by conducting a detailed clinical inter-view, assigning various questionnaires to complete at home, and asking clients to keep diaries and ratings of their anxiety experiences. By the second or third session they share this information with their clients and explain how to understand the person's anxiety from a cognitive perspective.

Assessment is the subject of this chapter (and was introduced in Chapter 1). We'll give you an overview of the principles behind a cognitive therapist's assessment meth-ods and also show you how to perform your own cognitive assessment if you're using this workbook on your own. Remember that only a qualified mental health profes-sional can accurately diagnose your anxiety problems, but by using the forms in this chapter you can gather enough information and understanding about your anxiety to allow you to work your way through this book toward achieving significant anxiety reduction.

Getting to Know Your Anxiety

By the end of this chapter you will be able to produce a cognitive behavior assessment of your anxiety problem; we're going to call it your *anxiety profile*. It will include information about your current problems and the thoughts, feelings, behaviors, and physical symptoms you experience during anxiety episodes. Your anxiety profile will sum up what triggers anxiety for you and how you respond to anxiety-producing situations, with a particular focus on your anxious thoughts, as well as details about how you tend to try to cope. **These aspects of anxiety are the main areas that you will explore using the worksheets in this chapter.**

Assessment—either by a therapist or via the self-help tools in this chapter—is critical to developing a "road map" for treatment.

"I Feel So Bad"

Whatever form your anxiety takes, your general anxiety level probably fluctuates from day to day. Tracking this daily level of general anxiety is important to determin-ing your progress in overcoming anxiety. If the workbook exercises are effective for you, one of the benefits obviously should be a reduction in your daily anxiety level. Beth was surprised to learn from her Rating Your Daily Anxiety record that she had more low-anxiety days than she realized. Use Worksheet 5.1 to track your generalized anxiety. **Make copies of the blank form so you can start using it today and continue using it as you work your way through this book.**

Try to complete the Rating Your Daily Anxiety record at the same time each day, preferably just before bedtime, since the anxiety rating is based on the average level of anxiety you experienced over the entire day. Try to use the full range of the 0–100 scale to capture the many variations that occur in generalized anxiety. Karen, for example, had a tendency always to rate her anxiety in the extreme (90–100). Yet it was clear from her descriptions that she experienced more variation in her generalized anxiety than her ratings reflected. So we worked on "recalibrating" her anxiety ratings so that 90 and above was reserved for unusual, extremely-high-anxiety days and her more usual anxiety days fell between 40 and 60. Mild anxiety was rated between 10 and 30.

Use the right-hand column to record anything that happened during the day that might have caused an increase in your general anxiety. You should record only those events, situations, or other triggers that are *directly* related to a spike in your anxiety level. Try to avoid second-guessing what you think might have caused an increase in your anxiety. Simply write down what occurred around the time you were feeling most anxious during the day. It is okay to leave this column blank if you didn't observe any triggers to your anxiety.

> Keep a record of your daily general anxiety level throughout the course of your cognitive intervention program.

⋛ Troubleshooting Tips ⋚

People often stop recording their daily anxiety level once they get into the more specific exercises in this workbook, which is unfortunate because it robs them of a useful tool for determining their progress in reducing anxiety. If you have a couple of bad days and feel discouraged about your progress, you can look back on the Rating Your Daily Anxiety record to see if overall you are making more progress than you think. Also, don't get too stressed about giving yourself a rating for the daily anxiety level. Remember, these numbers are not meant to be precise but rather a way of expressing whether your day was more or less anxiety-ridden.

"What Are My Triggers?"

Anxiety is highly reactive to situations. People tend to feel anxious in some situations but not in others, so a thorough evaluation of the external and internal triggers

Rating Your Daily Anxiety

Date: _____

Instructions: Use the rating scale below to record a number from 0 to 100 that indicates the average level of anxiety you experienced during the day. In the far right column, briefly describe any situations, events, experiences, or circumstances that occurred when you felt anxious that may have triggered the anxiety episode.

0_____50_____100

| Absolutely no anxiety, totally relaxed | Moderate or usual level of anxiety felt when in anxious state | Extreme, panic-stricken state that is unbearable and feels life-threatening |

Day of the Week/Date	Rating of Average Anxiety Level (0–100)	Anxiety Triggers Note any situations that increased your anxiety during the day.
1. Sunday		
2. Monday		
3. Tuesday		
4. Wednesday		
5. Thursday		
6. Friday		
7. Saturday		

of your anxiety is critical to addressing your particular problems. Worksheet 5.2 is designed to help you identify what triggers anxiety episodes for you. You may be so familiar with what triggers your anxiety that you could sit down and complete the form from memory. **However, it will be more accurate if you complete the form over several days, writing down the anxiety triggers associated with each anxiety episode as they occur. Make extra copies of this form, because if you're like most people you'll need to record many more than four anxiety-provoking situations.**

When recording the situation, keep your description brief. A simple phrase or three to four words will usually suffice. For example, triggers for Beth were "having to go to the supermarket because my husband is out of town," "attending 'meet the teacher' night at my children's school," "thinking about a staff meeting I have to attend at work in a few days," "feeling myself get hot and worrying that people will notice I'm getting anxious." Also try to think of your triggers more broadly. Often an external object or situation will trigger anxiety, but a certain physical sensation, thought, image, or memory may be the more specific direct trigger of the anxiety. Record any of these triggers in the "situation" column of the form. You should insert the date and time the anxiety episode occurred in the left-hand column.

Next provide a rating of the intensity of the anxiety episode. You can use the same 0–100 scale as for Worksheet 5.1. Also estimate the length of time your anxiety remains in the moderate-to-extreme range. Beth noted that it often took a couple of hours before her anxiety completely disappeared but that the duration of peak anxiety was only about 30 minutes.

The Identifying Your Anxiety Triggers form gives you a place for a thorough evaluation of the external and internal triggers that provoke your anxiety episodes.

In the final column, record your immediate coping response to feeling anxious. Most often this involves some form of escape or avoidance, but it could also include taking medication, asking others for reassurance, trying to relax yourself, and so on. A better understanding of your natural or automatic response to anxiety will provide key information for your treatment plan. Beth's most typical response to feeling anxious was to avoid people or escape from a social situation as quickly as possible.

⋛ Troubleshooting Tips ⋚

If you have trouble pinpointing your anxiety triggers after working with the form for a couple days, review your completed Worksheets 2.1 and 2.2 to recall what you initially recorded for situations, thoughts, and physical sensations that provoke your anxiety. If you're in treatment, your therapist may want to introduce you to the form by following the situational analysis guidelines presented in Chapter 5 of *Cognitive Therapy of Anxiety Disorders*.[5]

Identifying Your Anxiety Triggers

Instructions: Write down any situations, events, circumstances, thoughts, or physical sensations that may have triggered an anxiety episode. Very briefly describe the situation in column two, and in the third column rate the intensity of anxiety (0–100) and its duration (number of minutes). In the final column, note your immediate coping response to the situation—how you tried to control or reduce your anxiety.

Date/Time	Anxiety Triggers (i.e., situations, thoughts, physical sensations, events, expectations, etc.)	Anxiety Intensity (0–100) and Duration (minutes)	Coping Response to the Triggers
1.			
2.			
3.			
4.			

All Keyed Up

The physical symptoms of anxiety are often the most prominent and most disturbing feature of anxiety. There are important differences between people in how they feel physically when anxious and which symptoms bother them most. Consequently it's important to understand the physiological symptom profile associated with your anxiety experiences. Use Worksheet 5.3, Monitoring Your Physical Sensations, to gather detailed information on your physical symptoms of anxiety.

The Monitoring Your Physical Sensations form will be most helpful if you fill it in shortly after three separate anxiety episodes, since your physical symptoms may vary with each episode. In a very few words, describe the anxious situation and rate its intensity using a 0–100 scale (see the rating instruction key at the end of the form). Beside each symptom, rate how intensely you felt each physical sensation during the anxiety episode. In the next column briefly record any negative thoughts or interpretations about this symptom when it happens during an anxiety episode; what it is about the symptom that you don't like or that may actually frighten you when you're anxious. Place an asterisk beside the physical sensation that occurred first during the anxiety episode.

As an illustration, consider an anxiety episode that Beth had while stopping at the drug store earlier in the day to pick up her medication. The anxiety-provoking situation was "walking into the drug store and approaching the clerk at the prescription counter." She recorded the intensity of her anxiety as 75/100. The physical symptoms experienced included feeling warm/sweaty, hot flushes, muscle tension, chest discomfort, dry mouth, difficulty breathing, and lightheadedness. The most intense symptoms were feeling warm/sweaty (70/100), chest discomfort (65/100), and hot flushes (80/100), whereas muscle tension (40/100) and lightheadedness (25/100) were less intense. Her anxious interpretation of chest discomfort was "I must be quite anxious," whereas the most threatening interpretation was made to feeling warm/sweaty—"I am really feeling sweaty. What if it gets so bad the clerk notices that I'm sweating and wonders what's wrong with me?"—and the hot flush—"What if I start having a panic attack here in the store?" She interpreted muscle tension as a sign of stress but was concerned that the dry mouth would cause her difficulty with speaking to the clerk. Thus Beth learned from completing Worksheet 5.3 that "feeling warm/sweaty" and "hot flushes" were the physical symptoms that she considered most threatening and uncomfortable.

> Your physical symptom profile is critical information that you will later include in your overall anxiety profile and use to choose self-help exercises.

⋛ Troubleshooting Tips ⋚

Sometimes people end up checking only one or two physical symptoms of anxiety because they wait too long before completing Worksheet 5.3. This is a problem because it gives you

Monitoring Your Physical Sensations

Date: _____

Instructions: Write down any situations or experiences that cause an increase in your anxiety. Pay particular attention to whether you experience any of the bodily sensations listed on this form while you were in that situation. Rate how intensely you experienced the physical sensation using the 0–100 scale explained at the bottom of this worksheet. In the final column, briefly state what you disliked about each physical sensation you experienced or what was upsetting, even threatening, about the physical sensation. For you, what was so bad about having the physical sensation when you were feeling anxious?

1. ***Briefly describe anxious situation***: _____

   Anxiety level during episode (0–100 scale): _____

CHECKLIST OF PHYSICAL SENSATIONS DURING ANXIETY EPISODE

Physical Sensation	Rated Intensity of Physical Sensation	Negative Interpretation of Physical Sensation
Chest discomfort, pain, etc.		
Elevated heart rate		
Trembling, shaking		
Difficulty breathing		
Muscle tension		
Nausea, upset stomach		
Lightheaded, faint, dizzy		
Weak, unsteady		
Feeling warm, sweaty		
Chills, hot flushes		
Difficulty swallowing, choking sensation		
Dry mouth		
Other physical sensations: _____		

Intensity of Physical Sensations Scale: 0 = barely felt the sensation; 50 = strong sense of the sensation; 100 = dominant, overwhelming feeling.

2. ***Briefly describe anxious situation***: _____

   Anxiety level during episode (0–100 scale): _____

CHECKLIST OF PHYSICAL SENSATIONS DURING ANXIETY EPISODE

Physical Sensation	Rated Intensity of Physical Sensation	Negative Interpretation of Physical Sensation
Chest discomfort, pain, etc.		
Elevated heart rate		
Trembling, shaking		
Difficulty breathing		
Muscle tension		
Nausea, upset stomach		
Lightheaded, faint, dizzy		
Weak, unsteady		
Feeling warm, sweaty		
Chills, hot flushes		
Difficulty swallowing, choking sensation		
Dry mouth		
Other physical sensations: _____		

Intensity of Physical Sensations Scale: 0 = barely felt the sensation; 50 = strong sense of the sensation; 100 = dominant, overwhelming feeling.

(*cont.*)

3. ***Briefly describe anxious situation***: _____

    Anxiety level during episode (0–100 scale): _____

CHECKLIST OF PHYSICAL SENSATIONS DURING ANXIETY EPISODE

Physical Sensation	Rated Intensity of Physical Sensation	Negative Interpretation of Physical Sensation
Chest discomfort, pain, etc.		
Elevated heart rate		
Trembling, shaking		
Difficulty breathing		
Muscle tension		
Nausea, upset stomach		
Lightheaded, faint, dizzy		
Weak, unsteady		
Feeling warm, sweaty		
Chills, hot flushes		
Difficulty swallowing, choking sensation		
Dry mouth		
Other physical sensations: _____		

Intensity of Physical Sensations Scale: 0 = barely felt the sensation; 50 = strong sense of the sensation; 100 = dominant, overwhelming feeling.

an inaccurate picture of your anxiety experience. So be sure to complete the worksheet as close to an anxiety episode as possible, and don't skip over the last column. You may not interpret every physical symptom in an anxious way, but you undoubtedly will feel threatened or uncomfortable with at least one or two physical sensations. For each symptom ask yourself, "What is so upsetting about feeling this way?" "What is the worst that could happen to me because of this physical symptom?" or "Is there anything that scares me about this physical sensation when it hits me during an anxiety episode?" Finally make sure you write down your negative thoughts about the physical sensation when you're anxious and not after the fact, when you've calmed down.

Catching the Fear

You've already learned that core fear is the driving force behind anxiety and that this "core fear" consists of generating anxious thoughts about the likelihood and severity of future threat to yourself or loved ones. **Without question, the most important part of your anxiety assessment is determining the nature of your anxious mind.** Learning to identify your anxious or fearful thoughts is essential before you can take advantage of other cognitive and behavioral strategies to lower your anxiety level.

For this reason, you might want to spend a little extra time preparing to use Worksheet 5.4, Monitoring Your Anxious Thoughts. What threat or danger do you tend to think about when anxious? It's important to be aware of how you exaggerate the likelihood and severity of future threat when you're anxious. This tendency to overestimate the possibility and severity of bad outcomes is at the heart of your core fear. No doubt it occurs most strongly when you feel anxious, so learning to catch your exaggerated evaluations of threat (i.e., catastrophizing) during anxiety episodes is an important part of cognitive therapy.

Make multiple copies of the Monitoring Your Anxious Thoughts form because you will need to repeatedly practice identifying how you tend to think mainly about threat and danger in anxious situations. The goal is to increase your sensitivity to your automatic tendency to focus on the worst so you become better at countering such thinking. The cognitive therapy strategies discussed later in the workbook depend on your ability to identify your automatic anxious or threat-related thinking. The following are some questions you can ask yourself when anxious that may help you identify how you are thinking dangerously (i.e., catastrophizing):

■ "What am I thinking is the worst possible outcome of this situation?"

■ "What is my 'What if?' thinking in this anxious situation (e.g., what if my mind goes blank, what if I am having a heart attack, what if I have a panic attack, etc.)?"

Monitoring Your Anxious Thoughts

Date: _____

Instructions: Record your anxiety episodes in the first column and rate their intensity on the 0–100 scale. Next, write down the negative or threatening thoughts that went through your mind during the anxiety episode. In the final column, briefly describe what, for you, would be the worst imaginable outcome or negative consequence associated with this anxiety episode. You should record the "imagined catastrophe" even if you think it is highly unlikely. Try to fill in this form while you are in the anxious situation or as soon afterward as possible.

Anxiety Episode* (Briefly describe the anxious experience; its symptoms, situation, and outcome.)	Intensity of Anxiety (0–100 scale)	Threatening Thoughts (What personal negative consequences, threats, or dangers are you thinking about while experiencing this anxiety episode?)	Imagined Catastrophe (What's the worst outcome associated with this anxiety episode that you can imagine?)
1.			
2.			
3.			

*Mark an asterisk beside anxiety episodes that were full-blown panic attacks.

- "What am I thinking is the negative consequence for me in this situation?"
- "How am I thinking about the likelihood and severity of threat to me or others in this situation?"

It's important to distinguish the initial automatic threat or danger thought that occurs during peak anxiety from a much slower, more rational reevaluation of the anxious situation. Right now we're more concerned that you learn to identify your first thoughts about threat when you feel anxious. The following illustration might help explain the difference.

"Imagine for a moment that you are walking down a deserted street or country road by yourself and it is getting dark. Suddenly you hear a noise behind you. You immediately stiffen, your heart beats quickly, and you quicken your pace. Why this sudden surge of adrenalin? No doubt you instantly interpret the noise as a dangerous possibility: 'Could someone be approaching from behind who could cause me harm?' You turn around and there is no one there. Quickly you think to yourself 'No one is there, it must have been the wind, a squirrel, or my imagination.' It is this secondary thought, this reevaluation of the situation, that sticks in your mind. If later I asked you about your walk, you would remember a momentary twinge of fear and the later realization that 'nothing was there.' That first apprehensive thought that triggered the fear 'Is there an attacker behind me?' is lost to recall, instead replaced by your reasoned response to the situation."*

Previously you described a number of situations that cause you considerable anxiety (Worksheet 5.2). In these situations you would have had some initial apprehensive or danger-related thoughts that fueled your anxiety. It may be that now you can't remember what they are because you don't feel threatened at the moment and you're not in an anxiety-provoking situation. However, it's important to cognitive therapy that you discover the first threat-related thoughts; that is, that you learn to "catch your fear." We want to know what kick-starts the anxiety. If you're in treatment, it is likely your therapist will spend considerable time carefully going over your entries in Worksheet 5.4 to help you become better at catching that first threatening or danger-related thought or image during your anxiety episodes. In the last column, try to determine whether the thought or image of a more extreme, catastrophic outcome enters your mind when you are anxious. For example, can you trace your immediate anxious thinking to some ultimate worst-case scenario like succumbing to a deadly disease, being humiliated or ridiculed in front of people, or being left alone and destitute?

Table 5.1 lists some examples of threat-related thinking that represent core fears associated with common anxiety concerns. Use this table to guide you in discovering your own automatic anxious thoughts about impending threat or danger.

---

*From *Cognitive Therapy of Anxiety Disorders* by David A. Clark and Aaron T. Beck (p. 142).[5]

TABLE 5.1. **Examples of Anxious Situations and Their Associated Automatic Anxious Thoughts**

Anxiety-provoking situation	Automatic anxious thoughts or images (i.e., threat- or danger-focused thinking while anxious)
Anticipate meeting with supervisor at work	"What if she is angry at me and starts yelling? I'll get emotional and lose control. She'll lose respect for me, and I won't be able to face her again."
Son misses his curfew and is late returning the car on a Friday night	"What if he has been drinking and is involved in a terrible accident?"
Shopping in a crowded department store	"What if I start to feel anxious and get that trapped feeling? It could develop into a severe panic attack."
Can't get to sleep at night	"What if I can't fall asleep tonight? I'll be exhausted tomorrow and unable to work. If this continues, I could lose my job. After all, they are laying off people at work."
Have unexplained chest pain	"What if I am having a heart attack and I can't get to the hospital in time?"
Initiating a conversation with a stranger	"What if I get real nervous and my voice is shaky? He will think there is something wrong with me, that I must have an anxiety disorder."
Looking at your monthly bank statement	"We are just meeting our bills and no more. I can't seem to save any money. What if I can't save for retirement? I'll end up poor and destitute in my old age."

After monitoring her anxiety episodes and threat-related thinking for two weeks, Beth discovered her core fear. The anticipation of meeting people made her feel intense anxiety. She observed that during these anxious episodes her threat-related thinking went like this: "What if I start feeling hot and sweaty from stress and anxiety? People may notice that I'm perspiring and think there is something wrong with me." However, she was also able to capture more extreme catastrophic thinking: "My sweating may be so bad that I give off a body odor that is thoroughly disgusting to people standing close to me. I simply couldn't bear the embarrassment this would cause."

> Learning to recognize your initial automatic threat-related thoughts (i.e., tendency to catastrophize) is the first step in gaining some control over your anxiety experiences.

> ⋛ **Troubleshooting Tips** ⋚
>
> Many people have great difficulty identifying their more extreme, automatic threat-related thinking when feeling anxious. If this is happening to you, you're probably more focused on the physical symptoms of anxiety or how bad you feel. Practice asking yourself frequently during the day, "What am I thinking right now?" It may be easier to capture automatic threat-related thoughts when less anxious, so start with asking yourself "What uncomfortable thoughts am I having?" during less intense anxiety episodes and then work up to the more intense ones. Remember it is important to catch your automatic threat-related thoughts as close to the anxiety episode as possible, because later you'll forget them. Also you can review Chapter 2 and see what you entered in the core fear column of Worksheet 2.1. Then take another look at how you filled out Worksheets 3.1 and 3.2. This might remind you of the type of thinking you should look out for during anxiety episodes.

Thinking Mistakes

As you learned in Chapter 3, when we focus entirely on our thoughts of threat and danger, we often commit errors in logic that lead us to unrealistic, even irrational, conclusions. These cognitive errors contribute to our false assumption that some severe threat is highly likely to occur. **We've found that teaching people to become more aware of their thinking errors when feeling anxious can help them correct their faulty anxious thoughts and beliefs.** To record some examples of how you engage in thinking errors when feeling anxious, use Worksheet 5.5, Identifying Your Thinking Errors. Remind yourself of your automatic threat-related thinking by looking over Worksheet 5.4. Then ask yourself how the various errors listed on the left side of Worksheet 5.5 are present in your anxious thinking

> Becoming aware of your thinking errors is an important step in correcting faulty anxious thoughts and beliefs.

and enter them in the space provided on the form. **Make several copies of this form so you can fill it in periodically throughout this workbook to improve your ability to catch and correct the biases and errors that dominate anxious thinking.**

In fact you will want to review Worksheet 5.5 every time you work on correcting your anxious thinking so you will be able to pick out the cognitive errors and biases present in your anxious thinking. Beth, for example, really began to see that tunnel vision and emotional reasoning were dominant errors in her anxious thinking. When anxious, she would focus only on threat cues in social settings ("People are looking at me"—tunnel vision) and how uncomfortable she felt ("People must notice that

Identifying Your Thinking Errors

Date: _____

Instructions: Use this form to write down examples of your thinking errors when you feel anxious. Focus on how you are thinking when you are in anxious situations or anticipating the situation. Also focus on your most immediate threat-related thoughts rather than any secondary reconsideration of the situation.

Thinking Error	Examples of Your Anxious Thinking Errors
Catastrophizing	
Jumping to conclusions	
Tunnel vision	
Nearsightedness	
Emotional reasoning	
All-or-nothing thinking	

I'm anxious because I feel so uncomfortable"—emotional reasoning). Realizing that she made these errors helped Beth learn to correct her exaggerated thoughts of other people's negative evaluation.

> ### ⋛ Troubleshooting Tips ⋚
>
> If you have difficulty picking out the cognitive errors in your anxious thinking, a review of the different types of thinking errors in Table 3.2 might be helpful. Also it's sometimes easier to notice the cognitive errors in the way other people talk about issues. You can start by noting other people's cognitive errors and then gradually begin applying it to your own thinking about nonanxious concerns. After you've become good at picking out cognitive errors and biases in nonanxious thought, try applying it to your anxious way of thinking. It should be much easier to do after you practice identifying cognitive errors in the nonanxious thinking of yourself and others.

Pushing Back on Anxiety

Feeling anxious is horrible! In all our years of treating anxious patients, we have never met one person who said he or she liked the feeling of anxiety. Most people like to feel excited, and many seek out adventure and "the adrenaline rush," but no one seeks out anxiety. Since anxiety is such a highly distressing state, relief from anxiety is itself a positive, welcomed goal. For years psychologists have known that feeling relief or reduction from heightened anxiety is highly reinforcing.[27] It's no surprise, then, that anything that brings us even temporary relief from anxiety will be something we'll continue to do whenever we feel anxious, even if in the long term it causes the persistence of anxiety. Dick felt intense anxiety whenever he experienced an unexplained ache or pain. His automatic anxious thought was that something must be seriously wrong with his health, and then he would tend to catastrophize—wondering whether it could be cancer or some other deadly disease. He would immediately search the Internet for reassurance that the ache or pain was really something benign, like a sore muscle. In the short term he might feel some relief by finding some positive information, but in the long term his reassurance seeking made the anxiety worse by making him think that he had to take every ache and pain seriously.

When you feel anxious, you feel like you have no control—that the worst is about to happen and there is little you can do to stop it. So a natural response to that perceived loss of control is to try even harder to exert control. Robert Leahy, in his influential self-help book *Anxiety Free: Unravel Your Fears Before They Unravel You,* argues that a relentless effort to seize control is a basic element of fear and anxiety.[28] People with anxiety problems believe that the best defense against the worst thing happening is to take control. It is the belief that "if I am in control, I can avert the perceived threat or danger." So the person who is afraid of having a panic attack takes control by avoiding places that might cause panic. The individual who is anxious about his health might take control by excessively monitoring his body for signs that "all is not well" and then seek medical consultation. A person with social anxiety might try to conceal her anxiety in social situations. In each of these cases the person's control efforts are intended to avoid some imagined catastrophe like having a panic attack in public, contracting a deadly disease, or embarrassing herself in front of others.

There are three major problems with control in anxiety:

1. Creation of false control. The control you seek is unattainable because the fear is internally based; it is a thought, feeling, or sensation that remains no matter what you do or where you go. Therefore, any sense of control is merely temporary and creates only an illusion of safety. For example, if you were afraid of having a heart attack, you might work hard to avoid a racing heart rate even though there is no evidence that keeping your heart rate low is an effective way to reduce risk of cardiovascular disease (in fact, medical experts say the opposite—moderate exercise—is good for your heart).

2. Dependence on maladaptive control responses. Because you want immediate relief from anxiety, you will reach for control responses that produce a quick fix. Thus strategies like escape, avoidance, and seeking reassurance are used even though these strategies are responsible for the persistence of the anxiety problem. So the mantra in anxiety becomes *"long-term pain for short-term gain."*

3. Excessive preoccupation. The perceived need for control can quickly take over your life and become your primary daily goal. Decisions that involve meeting the basic demands of family, work, and community living are made based on what will minimize your anxiety and ensure a sense of comfort and security. In the end the need to control anxiety, to avert the worst possible outcome, can take over your life and greatly limit your ability to function. Robert Leahy notes that in the end attempts at control leave you feeling more out of control.[28]

What types of behavioral, emotional, and cognitive strategies do you use to push back anxiety—to try to reduce anxiety to a minimum and prevent some imagined worst-case scenario? Discovering your maladaptive coping responses to anxiety is an important part of cognitive intervention. Changing how you respond to anxiety is a critical goal in treatment. Worksheets 5.6 and 5.7 each present a list of common behavioral and cognitive strategies used to control anxiety. Read through each list and rate how often you employ each strategy when anxious and the perceived effectiveness of the strategy in reducing anxiety. If you have difficulty recalling your control responses, try completing these worksheets shortly after your anxiety episodes, with particular attention to how you automatically responded in that situation. Beth would

Behavioral Coping Checklist

Date: _____

Instructions: Below is a checklist of various ways that people tend to respond to anxiety. Please estimate how often you engage in each response **when you are anxious** and your impression of how well the strategy reduces or eliminates anxious feelings.

Scale Descriptions: What's your impression of how often you use this response when you feel anxious? [0 = never, 50 = half of the time, 100 = all the time]; What's your impression of its effectiveness in reducing your anxiety? [0 = not at all; 50 = moderately effective in reducing anxiety, 100 = completely eliminates my anxiety]

Behavioral and Emotional Responses	How Often (0–100 scale)	Effective in Reducing Anxiety (0–100 scale)
1. Try to physically relax (muscle relaxation, controlled breathing, etc.)		
2. Avoid situations that trigger anxiety		
3. Leave situations whenever I feel anxious		
4. Take prescription medication		
5. Seek reassurance and support from spouse, family, or friends		
6. Engage in a compulsive ritual (e.g., check, wash, count)		
7. Distract myself with activities		
8. Suppress my feelings (i.e., hold in my feelings)		
9. Use alcohol, marijuana, or other street drugs		
10. Get very emotional, tearful		
11. Have an anger outburst		
12. Become physically aggressive		

(cont.)

13. Speak or act more quickly in a hurried manner		
14. Become quiet, withdraw from others		
15. Seek medical/professional help (e.g., call therapist or GP; go to emergency room)		
16. Use Internet to chat with friend or obtain information		
17. Reduce physical activity level		
18. Rest, take a nap		
19. Try to find solution to the problem causing me anxiety		
20. Pray, meditate in an effort to reduce anxious feelings		
21. Have a smoke		
22. Have a cup of coffee		
23. Gamble		
24. Engage in pleasurable activity		
25. Eat comforting food (e.g., favorite junk food)		
26. Seek some place that makes me feel safe, not anxious		
27. Listen to relaxing music		
28. Watch TV or DVDs		
29. Do something that is relaxing (e.g., take a warm bath or shower, have a massage)		
30. Seek out a person who makes me feel safe, not anxious		
31. Do nothing, just let the anxiety "burn itself out"		
32. Engage in physical exercise (e.g., go to the gym, run)		
33. Read spiritual, religious, or meditative material (e.g., Bible, poetry, inspirational books)		
34. Go shopping (buy things)		

Identifying Your Cognitive Coping Checklist

Date: _____

Instructions: Below is a checklist of various ways that people try to control their anxious and worrisome thoughts. Using the rating scales below, please provide your impression of how often you engage in each response **when you are anxious** and whether you think the strategy is generally effective in reducing or eliminating anxiety.

Scale Descriptions: How often do you engage in this response when you feel anxious? [0 = never, 50 = half of the time, 100 = all the time]; When you engage in this cognitive strategy, generally how effectively does it reduce or eliminate anxiety? [0 = not at all; 50 = moderately effective in reducing anxiety, 100 = completely eliminates my anxiety]

Cognitive Control Response to Anxious Thinking	How Often (0–100 scale)	Effective in Reducing Anxiety (0–100 scale)
1. Deliberately try not to think about what is making me anxious or worried		
2. Tell myself that everything will be okay, will turn out fine		
3. Try to rationalize the anxiety; look for reasons why my anxious concerns might be unrealistic		
4. Try to distract myself by thinking about something else		
5. Try to replace the anxious thought with a more positive or comforting thought		
6. Make critical or negative remarks to myself about being anxious		
7. Tell myself simply to "stop thinking" like this		
8. Think a comforting phrase or prayer		
9. Ruminate on the anxious thought or worry; I keep going over in my mind what happened in the past or what could happen in the future		
10. When I start to feel anxious, I try to suppress the feelings so I don't look nervous or upset		

Because maladaptive control responses are an important contributor to the persistence of anxiety problems, letting go of these unhelpful strategies is an important goal of the workbook intervention.

often leave situations when anxious (escape), distract herself with activities, take an antianxiety pill, listen to relaxing music, or try to relax physically. However, only escaping anxious situations and taking medication seemed effective in reducing anxiety. Her cognitive control strategies included trying to rationalize the anxiety, think about something else, or critically tell herself not to be so stupid. None of these were effective in reducing anxious thoughts and feelings.

⸙ Troubleshooting Tips ⸙

Most people find it easier to identify their behavioral control strategies than the cognitive ones. If you have difficulty identifying your cognitive control strategies, start by observing the strategies you use to "not think about" distressing things that are not necessarily related to your anxiety concerns. What control strategies do you use to avoid unwanted thoughts? Then switch to your anxiety concerns and see whether you use the same control strategies to avoid your anxious thoughts. If you're in therapy, your therapist will want to review your responses to Worksheets 5.6 and 5.7.

"I'm So Worried"

In Chapter 3 we introduced worry as an important contributor to persistence of anxiety (see "Preparing for the Worst," pages 48–49). We suggest you review this section again as well as the list of anxious worries you recorded in the workbook. Once you have completed your review, you are ready to take the next step in discovering the nature of your worry. Worksheet 5.8, Identifying Your Worries, is designed to help you discover how worry is linked to your anxiety triggers and the initial automatic anxious thought about threat or danger. The form provides space for recording information about worry during several anxiety episodes.

First record the anxiety episode and rate its intensity as you've been doing on other worksheets in this chapter. Then write down any worries associated with the anxious episode in the final column. You may have worried about something related to the anxiety-provoking situation (e.g., anxious about meeting with your supervisor and worried that she might criticize your work performance) or you may be worried about the anxiety itself (e.g., that you have heart palpitations when you're anxious and worry these could eventually cause a heart attack).

One of Beth's major worries was the negative impact that her anxiety was having on her marriage. On her worksheet she recorded a recent anxiety episode in

Identifying Your Worries

Date: _____

Instructions: Record whether you have any worries associated with your anxiety. In the first column, briefly describe the anxiety episode and then rate the intensity of the anxiety on the 0–100 scale. In the third column, write down anything that worried you about the anxiety-provoking situation or about the anxiety itself. Also indicate how long the worry lasted (number of minutes or hours).

Anxiety Episode Briefly describe the anxious experience; its symptoms, situation, and outcome.	**Intensity of Anxiety** (0–100 scale)	**Worry Content** Is there anything that worries you about the situation or the effects of anxiety? Is there any negative consequence that worries you? How long did you worry?
1.		
2.		
3.		
4.		
5.		

Reprinted with permission from *Cognitive Therapy of Anxiety Disorders* by David A. Clark and Aaron T. Beck (p. 173). Copyright 2010 by The Guilford Press.

which she became quite anxious after her husband complained that they never go anywhere as a couple. After his complaint she experienced an intense period of anxiety (80/100), during which she felt tense, had hot flushes, and felt like she couldn't breathe properly. One worry theme focused on the anxious situation (her marriage): "What if Jeff loses patience with me and has an affair?" "How could I ever survive without him?" "I couldn't possibly raise these children as a single parent." The other worry theme focused on the negative effects of anxiety itself: "What if I never get over this anxiety?" "What if I become completely housebound and helpless?" "What if the anxiety robs me of everything?"

> Worry is the fuel thrown onto the "fires of anxiety" that intensifies the heat and endurance of the flame. Discovering how you worry during anxiety episodes is a final piece of the anxiety puzzle that is targeted for change in cognitive therapy.

⋛ Troubleshooting Tips ⋜

Review the section in Chapter 3 called "Preparing for the Worst" if you need a refresher on what constitutes worry. Worksheet 3.5 will show you what you recorded while reading that chapter as your anxious worries if you need a reminder to help you fill out Worksheet 5.8. If worry is a major problem in your anxiety, you will want to use the more detailed specialized worry forms in Chapter 11 to assess your worry experiences.

Your Anxiety Profile

Now that you've gathered detailed information on your anxious mind, you're ready to build an outline of your anxiety that will guide your cognitive therapy over the next three chapters. Use Worksheet 5.9 to put together your Anxiety Profile before proceeding to the next chapter. Following the blank worksheet is a filled-out example for Beth, the 36-year-old mother introduced at the beginning of this chapter. The instructions below explain how to use the worksheets you filled out in this chapter and in Chapter 3 to compile your Anxiety Profile.

I. Main Anxiety Triggers

Turn to your completed Worksheet 5.2 and use what you recorded there to list external situations and circumstances, as well as possible thoughts or physical sensations that trigger your anxiety episodes, at the top of your Anxiety Profile.

II. Evaluation of Threat and Danger

Next complete the various entries in the "Evaluation of Threat and Danger" box:

- **Use Worksheet 5.3** to help you summarize the physical symptoms you typically experience when anxious as well as any negative interpretation you make of these symptoms.

- **Use Worksheet 5.4** to fill in your automatic anxious thoughts that involve an overestimate of the probability and severity of personal threat or danger (i.e., how you tend to catastrophize when anxious, think about terrible things happening to you or loved ones).

- **Next, use Worksheet 5.5** to list the typical cognitive errors or mistakes that are evident in your anxious thinking.

- **Now turn back to Worksheet 3.3** to find the items that you strongly or completely agreed with to identify your core beliefs about your intolerance for anxiety and its consequences. What do you believe are the negative consequences of anxiety or its effects on you? Why is it so important that you control or reduce anxiety? What do you believe about your ability to tolerate being anxious?

III. Coping and Anxiety Control Responses

The third category in the Anxiety Profile deals with your deliberate coping strategies—your efforts to control anxiety, to reduce its intensity, and to minimize its negative effects in your life. How would you describe the coping strategies you use to deal with your anxious concerns?

- **Go back to Worksheet 3.2** and write down your most prominent thoughts of helplessness when anxious. How do you see yourself when it comes to coping with anxiety? At one time did you think of yourself as able to cope with considerable stress and anxiety? How has this changed as a result of your anxiety experiences? What types of self-critical thoughts do you now have when you are feeling anxious?

- **Now turn back to Worksheet 3.4** to list your avoidance patterns: situations, thoughts, feelings, or physical sensations you try to avoid to reduce the possibility of an anxiety episode.

- **Review the list of behavioral and cognitive safety-seeking strategies in Chapter 3 (pages 46–47)** to record your most prominent safety-seeking strategies; that is, the things you do to minimize anxiety and reestablish a state of calm, security, and comfort in your life.

Your Anxiety Profile

Instructions: Based on your answers to the exercises in Chapters 3 and 5, complete each of the sections in this flowchart. This will be used to set treatment goals and guide your cognitive therapy sessions.

I. MAIN ANXIETY TRIGGERS
(i.e., situations, thoughts, sensations, expectations)

1. _____

2. _____

3. _____

4. _____

5. _____

II. EVALUATION OF THREAT AND DANGER

Physical sensations: _____

_____

Evaluation of physical sensations: _____

_____

Automatic thoughts about threat, danger, and catastrophe (core fear): _____

_____

Typical thinking errors (mistakes): _____

_____

Beliefs about anxiety: _____

_____

(*cont.*)

III. DELIBERATE COPING RESPONSES

Helplessness (vulnerability) thoughts: _____

_____

_____

Avoidance patterns: _____

_____

_____

Safety seeking: _____

_____

_____

Other coping responses: _____

_____

_____

Anxious worry: _____

_____

_____

Beth's Anxiety Profile

I. MAIN ANXIETY TRIGGERS

1. *Public places such as being in a supermarket, large restaurant, shopping mall, movie theater, etc.*

2. *Anticipating a social event like the end-of-week staff meeting*

3. *Having a conversation with an unfamiliar person*

4. *Feeling hot and uncomfortable, especially around other people*

5. *Remembering a social interaction I had with a person at work last week*

II. EVALUATION OF THREAT AND DANGER

Physical sensations: *muscle tension, hot flushes, sweaty, difficulty breathing, lightheadedness, dry mouth, chest discomfort*

Evaluation of physical sensations: *chest discomfort was a sign of mounting anxiety; feeling hot and sweaty was disturbing because people could see my anxiety and possibly be disgusted by my body odor; hot flushes were interpreted as a sign of an impending panic attack*

Automatic thoughts of threat, danger and catastrophe (core fear): *People will notice that I'm anxious and wonder what's wrong with me; they will find me disgusting because I am sweating so much; I'm embarrassing myself with this filthy sweating.*

Typical thinking errors (mistakes): *catastrophizing about sweating; tunnel vision* [can only think about being anxious when around people]; *jump to conclusions* [quick to assume she is embarrassing herself]; *emotional reasoning* [if she feels a little anxious, then she is about to lose control and really embarrass herself]

Beliefs about anxiety: *I can't stand feeling anxious; if I feel anxious around people, then I am more likely to embarrass myself; I can't carry on a sensible conversation when I'm anxious; I should be able to feel calm and relaxed around people.*

(cont.)

III. DELIBERATE COPING RESPONSES

Helplessness (vulnerability) thoughts: _that I am emotionally weak and easily overwhelmed; that I lack social skills and so I'm more likely to embarrass myself; that people notice I'm awkward and self-conscious in social settings and so this draws attention to me_

Avoidance patterns: _avoid most public places; limit social interaction to family and one or two old friends; avoid situations where I may be the focus of attention_

Safety-seeking responses: _carry medication whenever I leave home; wear heavy clothes to conceal perspiration; try to form a pleasant image whenever I feel anxious ("going to my safe place")_

Other coping responses: _try to convince myself I haven't done anything embarrassing_ [rationalization]; _try to think about anything but anxiety_ [distraction]; _tell myself I'm being stupid for feeling anxious_ [self-criticizing]

Anxious worry: _worried that Jeff might leave me; worried that my anxiety will get worse and I'll lose my job; worried that my very shy 8-year-old daughter will develop an anxiety problem like her mother_

■ **Now use Worksheets 5.6 and 5.7** to list other coping responses you use when feeling anxious.

■ **Use Worksheet 5.8** to fill in the things you tend to worry about when anxious.

If you are seeing a cognitive therapist, it will be important to discuss with her your responses to Worksheet 5.9. Your work on developing a cognitive self-assessment will be very helpful to your therapist's more detailed assessment that might be based on outlines such as Appendix 5.11 in *Cognitive Therapy of Anxiety Disorders.*[5] Your cognitive therapist may also want to work collaboratively with you on your cognitive profile to help you pinpoint the thought processes most critical to the maintenance of your anxiety problems. If you're reading the workbook on your own, you will want to refer back to Worksheet 5.9 frequently as you work through the remaining chapters. Your Anxiety Profile will be an important guide, informing you where changes need to be made to overcome your problems with anxiety.

You develop a personal "anxiety profile" before starting an intervention program to ensure that cognitive and behavioral strategies target the specific contributors to your persistent anxiety.

Now that you have worked through the cognitive perspective and developed your own Anxiety Profile, we will use this information in the next three chapters to construct your cognitive therapy program—or, to put it another way, to develop a unique mental fitness exercise plan that will help you win the struggle over anxiety.

CHAPTER SUMMARY

■ Assessment is an important element of cognitive therapy. It provides a "road map" for tailoring the cognitive therapy interventions discussed in the next two chapters to the unique features of your anxiety.

■ Repeated examples of the triggers, physical symptoms, core anxious thinking, and thinking errors that characterize your everyday anxiety experiences are necessary to developing a good understanding of the cognitive basis of anxiety.

■ A critical evaluation of your tolerance for anxiety and how you try to control anxiety through escape, avoidance, and safety-seeking strategies is needed to fully understand your anxiety experiences.

■ Because most anxiety episodes are characterized by excessive worry, discovering the nature of your worry is another key aspect of assessment.

■ Worksheet 5.9 is used to construct your own Anxiety Profile based on the information you provided in the rating forms, structured diaries, and other worksheets in Chapters 3 and 5.

6

Transforming the Anxious Mind

At age 23 Philip was unemployed and living with his parents, and his hopes of getting out on his own were dwindling rapidly because his life seemed wrecked by anxiety. He had received a B.A. a year ago and was trying to get into law school but hadn't done well on the LSAT the first time and was having great difficulty studying to take it a second time. The pressure on him felt enormous—his father was a lawyer and his siblings had all gotten into law or medical school, and everyone in the family expected Philip to follow in their footsteps.

Philip felt keyed up and on edge much of the day. Every day he woke up feeling uneasy, as if something bad was about to happen, and also exhausted since anxiety kept disrupting his sleep. During the day he had a churning sensation in his stomach and had difficulty concentrating when he tried to study. His anxiety had occurred only occasionally at first, but in the last few months it had worsened to the point where he felt anxious practically all the time. He rarely went out but couldn't concentrate on studying, so he spent most of the day surfing the Web or watching movies.

Philip's anxiety had become incapacitating and was threatening to derail his career aspirations. Instead of focusing on the steps he needed to take to achieve his goal of attending law school, his mind reeled with worries about the future: "I'm losing my focus; I can't remember anything." "I don't understand what I'm studying." "I'll never do well on the LSAT." "I'll go into the exam and freeze." "I'll end up with such a low score, I'll never get into law school." "I can't even fill out the law school applications." "I don't know what to say about myself in the application; what if the admissions committee thinks my application sounds stupid?" "I'm going to end up alone and working at a fast food restaurant." "I'll be such a disappointment and embarrassment to my family." "I'll never be happy and end up one of those pathetic losers you read about in the news." This thinking was a driving force in Philip's anxiety and became a type of self-fulfilling prophecy, causing him to act in a way that could eventually lead to his most feared outcome. Philip's therapist focused directly on his worry. Helping him change his catastrophic thoughts about future failure reduced Philip's generalized anxiety and improved his ability to study for the law exams.

This chapter will help you do the same: change the thinking that is fueling your anxiety so you can reduce it to normal levels and minimize its damaging effects on your life. Chapter 7 will help you change anxiety-related behavior. In cognitive therapy we often work on anxiety-inducing thoughts first because this is good preparation for doing behavioral exercises, which people with anxiety often find more difficult and challenging. In this book, in fact, **we want you to read through Chapters 6 and 7 once without doing the exercises. Then turn to Chapter 8 to formulate an Anxiety Work Plan. Finally, return to the exercises in Chapters 6 and 7, working your way through them in order according to your plan and adding a new exercise every week or 10 days so that you are continuing to practice some old cognitive skills while adding new ones to work on.** You'll be working with all the information you gathered for your Anxiety Profile at the end of the preceding chapter, so be sure to have your filled-out Worksheet 5.9 handy once you actually start working with the exercises. The strategies you learn here will build on everything you learned in Chapter 3 about the anxious mind.

From Anxious Thinking to Normalized Thinking

If you've ever had a computer virus, you know that, once activated, the virus can quickly take over the operation of your computer. Clinical anxiety is a lot like a computer virus. Once activated, fear takes over so you think, feel, and behave in ways that end up perpetuating the anxiety. **The goal of cognitive therapy is to deactivate, or turn off, the fear program and return you to a normal state of functioning. This is achieved by transforming or changing your anxious thoughts and beliefs.**

Remember: Change the way you think about your anxious concerns and you will change your anxiety experience.

The diagram below illustrates this shift in thinking.

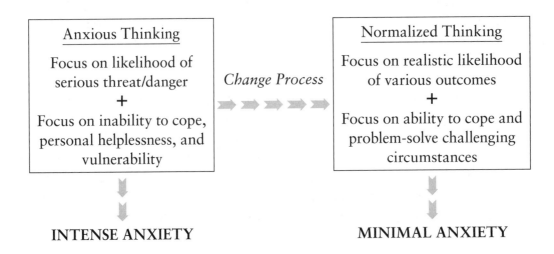

Using the exercises in this chapter, you'll work on transforming your anxious thinking that leads to intense anxiety to more normalized thinking that characterizes minimal anxiety. We'll follow the cognitive perspective on anxiety that you've been learning about throughout this book. Below you'll find a graphic summary of the specific features of anxious thinking targeted in this chapter. You have learned about these characteristics of anxious thinking both through our explanations in previous chapters and through your personal self-observation from doing the exercises:

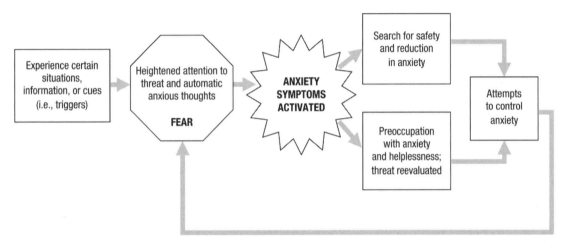

The anxious mind.

Reprinted with permission from *Cognitive Therapy of Anxiety Disorders* by David A. Clark and Aaron T. Beck (p. 193). Copyright 2010 by The Guilford Press.

As shown in the diagram, the first thing that happens is that some trigger activates the fear program. However, it's the next step, the heightened attention to the automatic thoughts of threat and danger, that really turns on the anxiety symptoms: You overestimate the likelihood and the severity of the perceived threat, you assume you're helpless, and you underestimate your safety. Combined, these automatic thoughts keep anxiety going. Whenever Philip thought about studying for his law exams, he would think, "This is hopeless; I'm not taking anything in" (helplessness assumption), "There is no way I'll get a good score" (high threat probability), "I'll end up doing worse than the first time I took the exam" (exaggerated threat severity), and "I've made absolutely no progress since I started studying a few weeks ago" (ignores safety information).

The objective of cognitive interventions is to correct these four aspects of anxious thinking, summarized in Table 6.1: the tendency to assume the very worst outcome is likely to happen (1 and 2), that if it did happen you would not be able to deal with it (3), and that threat and danger are more likely than safety (4).

Philip's anxious thinking was corrected so that he began to think "I am taking

TABLE 6.1. **Four Aspects of Anxious Thinking Targeted in Cognitive Therapy**

Term	Definition	Examples
1. High threat likelihood	Thinking that a bad outcome is more likely to happen than is realistically true.	• "I'll probably have a panic attack." • "I'll probably say something embarrassing in the meeting." • "People probably think I'm really weird and so would rather not have to interact with me." • "The company is downsizing; I'll probably get a pink slip soon."
2. Exaggerated threat severity	Thinking about the very worst outcome happening.	• "I could have such a severe panic attack that I'll end up going to the emergency room." • "It will be one of the most humiliating experiences in my life." • "I'll never find love and will end up living a lonely, miserable life." • "I'll lose my job and be unemployed for a long time, given the recession."
3. Helplessness assumptions	Thinking that I can't cope or deal with a future difficulty.	• "I can't handle intense anxiety." • "I don't know what to say in meetings." • "I have no confidence in myself; I'm careless and frequently make mistakes." • "I have extremely poor job search skills; I make terrible first impressions in job interviews."
4. Underestimate safety	Failing to notice safety aspects of situations.	• Fails to notice that anxiety is less severe than last time he was in a public place. • Fails to notice that work colleagues at the meeting are friendly and supportive. • Fails to remember the times when she was invited to join in on a conversation. • Ignores evidence that the company is finished with the current round of employee cuts.

in more information than I initially assumed" (increased self-confidence), "I am more likely to improve my LSAT score with this extra studying than I am to do worse" (corrected probability estimate), "I'm more likely to do only slightly better the second time than to actually do worse on the exam" (modified severity estimate), and "I may have wasted a lot of time procrastinating, but I'm better off in my exam preparation now than I was a few weeks ago" (better processing of safety information). Philip shifted toward normalized thinking by using eight cognitive strategies for anxiety reduction described in this chapter. We've labeled them "steps" to help you work through the exercises in a logical fashion, but they are all different parts of the cognitive approach. You will combine these steps and use them together to produce a concerted cognitive strategy, or Anxiety Work Plan (see Chapter 8), for reducing your anxious thinking.

Step 1: Normalizing from the start
Step 2: Catching automatic anxious thoughts
Step 3: Gathering evidence
Step 4: Doing a cost–benefit analysis
Step 5: Decatastrophizing the fear
Step 6: Correcting cognitive errors
Step 7: Generating alternative perspectives
Step 8: Practicing the normalization approach

You will notice that the exercises in this chapter mainly target the Evaluation of Threat and Danger part of your Anxiety Profile. So as you apply these exercises to your anxiety, you will want to structure them around the anxious thoughts, beliefs, and cognitive errors you identified in this section of your Anxiety Profile.

Cognitive interventions focus on transforming the anxious mind by recalibrating automatic threat and danger cognitions so they are more realistic, strengthening your confidence in your ability to cope with anxious concerns, and improving your recognition of the safe and benign aspects of situations that make you feel anxious.

Step 1: Normalizing from the Start

To change your anxious thinking, first it's important to know what you *should* be thinking: "If my thinking is faulty or exaggerated when I'm anxious, then what should I be thinking in this situation?"

As we've said, everyone has anxiety, so it's impossible to live without feeling anxious from time to time. Your goal should be to reduce anxiety, not eliminate it. So reminding yourself how you think when normally anxious can be very helpful in changing your faulty or incorrect thinking when intensely anxious. Everyone can remember being nervous before making a speech, writing an exam, meeting someone new, going to a job interview, anticipating a medical procedure, and the like. The number of things that we could be anxious about is endless! In the following spaces, list five things that happened in the last few months where you felt some brief but fairly mild anxiety or worry.

1. _____

2. _____

3. _____

4. _____

5. _____

Now take one of these normal anxiety experiences and complete Worksheet 6.1, the Normalization Chart. Based on the picture of anxious thinking in the diagram "The Anxious Mind" and Table 6.1, compare how you think when anxiety is normal and how you think when anxiety is severe or pathological. Reminding yourself how you think when you have normal anxiety can help when correcting the faulty thinking associated with intense anxiety. **Ask yourself, "How could I think more normally about my anxious concern?"** For example, what would be a more normal way to think about spontaneous heart palpitations, shortness of breath, speaking up at a meeting, worrying that you said something insensitive to another person or whether your spouse still loves you? From your Normalization Chart you can see that you can think normally about anxiety when it's low, so now the challenge is to apply the same way of thinking to when you have intense anxiety. A filled-out example for Philip follows the blank form.

You can think more realistically about anxious concerns by generating a good description of "normal anxious thinking" and referring to it whenever something triggers your anxiety. Practicing this will help you reach the goal of thinking this way whenever you experience an episode of intense anxiety.

⦚ Troubleshooting Tips ⦚

If you need to refresh your memory about your anxious concerns to fill out Worksheet 6.1, review your Worksheets 2.2, 3.1, and 5.2 for ideas.

Normalization Chart

Instructions: In the space provided, record an example of experiencing normal anxiety and then your main anxious concern. Briefly describe how you think when you experience normal anxiety versus when you experience problematic anxiety. We have broken anxious thinking into its various components described in Table 6.1.

1. Example of normal anxious experience: _____

_____

_____

2. My problematic anxious concern is: _____

_____

_____

Types of Cognitions	Normal Anxious Thinking	Problematic Anxious Thinking
Likelihood How likely is the negative outcome?		
Severity How severe is the negative outcome?		
Helplessness How helpless or unable do you feel to cope with the possible negative outcome?		
Underestimated Safety What might be safe or benign about this concern that you are overlooking?		

Philip's Normalization Chart

1. Example of normal anxious concern: _Last year I had to make a presentation in a fourth-year seminar course; I felt anxious about doing the presentation but prepared for it anyway and was able to give the presentation even though I felt very anxious at the time._

2. My problematic anxious concern is: _feeling anxious and worried about studying for law entrance exam and applying to law schools_

Types of Cognitions	Normal Anxious Thinking	Problematic Anxious Thinking
Likelihood How likely is the negative outcome?	_I always get nervous making presentations, and it seems to turn out okay. Lots of people get nervous making speeches._	_I just know I won't do well on the law exam. I can't even imagine how this could possibly have a good outcome._
Severity How severe is the negative outcome?	_I can still make a pretty good presentation even if I am feeling nervous. I may not get the highest grade in the class, but I'll do okay. It's not worth that much, so it won't affect my course grade even if I don't do as well as I wanted._	_My life is ruined. Without a good score on the law entrance exam, I'll never get into law school. I'm going to end up a real loser, an embarrassment to myself and my family._
Helplessness How helpless or unable do you feel to cope with the possible negative outcome?	_I've given presentations before when I was nervous, and I can do it again. Sure, the feelings are uncomfortable, but I can still get my points across in a presentation._	_I don't know what's wrong with me. I can't remember anything that I am studying. I am completely incapable of doing the LSAT. It's defeated me._
Underestimated Safety What might be safe or benign about this concern that you are overlooking?	_I've got my PowerPoint slides, and I've made some notes for myself. I can use these as a guide that will get me through the presentation even though I feel anxious. This way I have some aids to help me if my mind goes blank due to anxiety._	_I've made no progress in studying for this exam. I'm completely wasting time. The only solution is to quit so I can end the agony I feel._

Self-Help Exercise 6.1.
Normalizing Initial Thoughts

On a 3" × 5" index card, write down how you could think in a "normally anxious way" about your main anxious concern. Carry this card with you at all times. When your anxious concern returns, immediately review your *normal anxiety card*. If you have multiple anxious concerns, complete a normal anxiety card for each concern. You could also enter these statements into a smartphone or other mobile device.

Philip's normal anxiety card when worrying about the LSAT:

At this point I still have quite a few months to study for the law exam. I could do worse the next time I take the exam, but I could also do better. The future cannot be known, and I will be better prepared for the exam the next time because I will have studied more than the first time. I've always done well on exams in the past and have surprised myself with how much I remember even when I've been anxious. Failing to get into law school is not the end of the world. Lawyers are not the happiest, most fulfilled people in the world. I really can imagine myself living a fulfilled, satisfied life doing something different. Besides, I just took a practice exam, and I was surprised at how well I did despite having not studied much in the last month. So I'll give this one last try and then adjust my life to the outcome.

Step 2: Catching Automatic Anxious Thoughts

Part of the reason we get trapped in our catastrophizing thoughts is they occur so automatically that our anxious mind has taken over before we realize it. **So in cognitive therapy we teach people how to "catch automatic anxious thinking" so they can slow down enough to evaluate and correct those thoughts.** This second step in transforming the anxious mind, then, involves learning a new cognitive skill: consciously and intentionally identifying your exaggerated thoughts of threat and danger earlier and earlier in the anxiety cycle.

Like any other skill, learning to catch automatic anxious thoughts takes a lot of practice. It will come easier to some people, a bit harder to oth-

Use the Threat Assessment Diary to master your ability to catch automatic catastrophic thoughts of threat and danger during anxiety episodes. This will slow down your automatic thinking and reduce the feeling of uncontrollability that accompanies anxiety episodes.

ers. Regardless of your starting point, everyone who suffers from anxiety will need to practice this skill and will be able to improve his or her thought-monitoring skills. You'll be using a copy you've already made of Worksheet 5.4 to record your automatic anxious thoughts. Then you'll use a new one that allows you to go out into your daily life and write down your experience, broken down into the four main targets of cognitive therapy: exaggerated likelihood of threat, exaggerated severity of threat, assumed helplessness, and underestimation of safety.

Self-Help Exercise 6.2. Thought Monitoring

We suggest a two-step process for learning to catch your core anxious thoughts:

1. **Begin with Worksheet 5.4, Monitoring Your Anxious Thoughts,** and for a week or so record your automatic thoughts about threat every time you have a significant anxiety episode. The following are some questions you can ask yourself to catch your automatic fearful thinking:

   - "What is the first thing that went through my mind when I started to feel anxious?"
   - "What am I afraid of? What is the worst possible outcome, the catastrophe in this situation?"
   - "What concerns me most about this situation or how I am feeling?"

2. **Next use Worksheet 6.2, Threat Assessment Diary,** to break down the exaggerated threat and danger cognitions into their core features. **You should make multiple copies of this form. You will need to focus exclusively on learning to catch anxious thinking with this form for 1 to 2 weeks and then afterward use it often for as long as you are working on the skills described in this workbook.**

⋛ Troubleshooting Tips ⋜

Sometimes people are reluctant to monitor their anxious thoughts, fearing it will make them worse because they'll be paying even more attention to their fearful thoughts. This might be a legitimate concern if all you did was simply write down your anx-

Threat Assessment Diary

Anxious, Threat-Related Thought	Likelihood Estimate How likely is the negative, threatening outcome?	Severity Estimate How severe is the negative, threatening outcome?	Helplessness How much do you feel helpless or unable to cope with the possible negative, threatening outcome?	Underestimated Safety What might be safe or benign about this concern that you are overlooking?
1.				
2.				
3.				
4.				

ious thoughts (a process called "journaling"). But this self-monitoring phase is only an intermediate step, though an important one. You can't benefit from the more advanced strategies until you've mastered the skill of catching your automatic anxious thoughts. Identifying your anxious thoughts and images, writing them down, and then reading over your entries will slow down your catastrophic thinking and enrich your understanding of your anxiety episodes.

If you feel too anxious during an episode to write anything down, try to fill out the form as soon afterward as you can. If you're feeling a little overwhelmed with the detailed information required in Worksheet 6.2, you could return to Worksheet 5.4 and practice with it a little longer. However, you will want to progress to using Worksheet 6.2, because correcting exaggerated thinking about the likelihood and severity of threat is an important cognitive intervention.

Step 3: Gathering Evidence

You may have watched at least one episode of the TV program *CSI* on crime scene investigation. One of the most popular phrases in the show is "What does the evidence say?" or "Let the evidence speak." What if you took the same approach to your anxious thoughts of threat and danger and looked for evidence that confirms or denies the imagined danger? If you have panic attacks, what's the evidence your heart palpitations could be a heart attack? If you have social anxiety, what is the evidence that you're humiliating yourself in front of others?

Taking the perspective of a detective questioning your own anxious thoughts and beliefs is extremely difficult. Most people get caught up in the emotion and abandon their reasoning skills. But this is an important cognitive therapy skill that can be used to reduce anxious thoughts and beliefs. Evidence gathering is a major cognitive therapy strategy for correcting the exaggerated thoughts about threat and danger that are responsible for your anxiety.

Questioning anxious thoughts and beliefs through evidence gathering is a key clinical skill in cognitive therapy for correcting the exaggerated thoughts of threat and personal helplessness, which are important contributors to your anxiety. It takes repeated daily practice to perfect the use of evidence gathering as an effective anxiety-reduction tool.

Angela, for example, had intrusive anxious thoughts about death and dying. Whenever she had these thoughts, she would seek reassurance from her husband that she was really healthy and would not die from some deadly disease. These thoughts caused so much anxiety that Angela started to believe maybe she was destined for an early death; that somehow being so preoccupied with death was a bad omen. She knew her thinking was illogical, but that didn't seem to make her feel any better. She became more and more anxious every time she experienced the "death thoughts." Using the Threat Assessment Diary, Angela's cognitive therapist first clarified her core fear—"that thinking about death is threatening, dangerous because it might make it more likely to come true." Then Angela was asked to gather evidence for and against the belief that "thinking about death makes it more likely to happen."

Self-Help Exercise 6.3.
Gathering the Evidence

Developing an effective evidence-gathering tool takes time and repetition. **Make multiple copies of Worksheet 6.3, Gathering Evidence, since the evidence you gather for one anxious concern may take up one or more pages. You want to make sure you have copies of the form to use for other anxious concerns.**

1. Begin by completing Worksheet 6.3 when you're not feeling anxious. On the first line, write down your main automatic anxious or catastrophizing thought.

2. **Then, over the next week, carry the form with you.** Add to the evidence for or against the threat-related anxious thought every time you experience something that reminds you "why I should be afraid of the anxious concern" and "why I should not be afraid of the anxious concern." The goal is to generate as much evidence as possible for and against the anxious thought. After you have generated your list, circle the evidence that you find most convincing.

3. Once you've obtained many pieces of evidence for and against your core anxious thought, **rate the likelihood and severity of the outcome based on the realistic evidence you collected.** *Remember, these ratings are based on the evidence you gathered and not on how you feel.*

On his evidence-gathering form, Philip wrote down the anxious thought "I can't study for the LSAT because I can't concentrate or remember anything" (item 1). He then listed the following evidence for the anxious thought:

■ He had not studied in the last several weeks (*evidence of worst outcome*).

■ When he tried to study, he became very anxious (*evidence of worst outcome*).

Gathering Evidence

Date: _____

Write down the anxious thought about threat or danger you are testing: _____

Evidence for Threatening Thought	Evidence against Threatening Thought
What is the evidence that the threat is highly likely to occur? What evidence do you have for the worst outcome? What's the evidence that you can't cope with the negative outcome?	What is the evidence that the threat is not as likely as you think? What is the evidence that the outcome will be only mildly unpleasant? Is there any evidence that you may be able to cope with the negative outcome? Is there any evidence that the situation is safer than you think?
1.	1.
2.	2.
3.	3.
4.	4.

* Use additional pages to list evidence for and against.

Based only on the gathered evidence (and not on how you feel), rate how likely it is that the threat will occur from 0% (won't happen) to 100% (certain): _____ %

Based only on the gathered evidence (and not on how you feel), rate the severity of the most likely outcome from 0% (not at all severe) to 100% (most severe I can imagine): _____ %

- He was able to study for only 20 minutes at a time even when he felt less anxious (*evidence of not coping*).

- Every time he quizzed himself after studying even a little he would get wrong answers (*evidence of high likelihood of not remembering*).

Philip found it tough to search for evidence contrary to his anxious thought but eventually came up with the following:

- When he decided to take out his books and just read a few pages of study material, he was surprised that he was able to actually read a few pages when he didn't put pressure on himself to memorize the material (*evidence against worst outcome*).

- Philip admitted that in the past he would get more questions right than wrong when he quizzed himself. Clearly, he was remembering some of the material (*evidence against worst outcome*).

- When taking undergraduate courses, Philip had a great ability to cram for exams and actually retain a large amount of material in a short period of time (*evidence of ability to cope*).

- He found he could study for the LSAT better if he kept his study time to 20-minute periods with plenty of breaks in between (*evidence of safety, ability to cope*).

- Even when he was highly anxious while studying, it was not true that he remembered absolutely nothing (*evidence against likelihood and severity of worst outcome*).

Based just on the evidence, Philip admitted that the probability of not remembering anything was really 25% and that a much less serious outcome (20%)—not being able to remember as much material as he would like—was more likely. He agreed that the evidence indicated his anxious thinking was clearly exaggerated. Then he completed the evidence-gathering form every time he became anxious about studying because he was thinking that he wasn't taking anything in. Reviewing the evidence against the thought on the form, he would correct his faulty anxious thought by reminding himself that the anxious thought was an exaggeration, a false notion about threat (i.e., the imagined negative effects of his struggle to study).

⸕ Troubleshooting Tips ⸕

If you're having difficulty with evidence gathering, use the questions under the column headings in Worksheet 6.3 to guide your efforts. Notice that these questions correspond to the breakdown we used in Worksheet 6.2. In fact, it may be helpful to review your information in Worksheet 6.2 to better target your evidence-gathering efforts in Worksheet 6.3. Also, you need to be realistic about the benefits of evidence gathering. Don't expect your anxious thinking to disappear now that you are disputing it with contrary evidence. Evidence gathering is a strategy for **repeatedly correcting anxious thinking when it occurs!** That's why it's so important to repeatedly practice responding to your anxious episodes by **questioning, questioning, questioning** the anxious thoughts. Keep asking yourself, "But what is the evidence that I am exaggerating the probability and severity of the situation and underestimating my ability to cope or that I'm ignoring the safety of the situation?"

Step 4: Doing a Cost–Benefit Analysis

People who struggle with anxiety often develop ways of responding that worsen their anxiety in the long run. They come to believe that worry, avoidance, reassurance seeking, and the like are the only way to deal with anxiety. Or they accept their exaggerated beliefs in threat and danger as the only way to respond. One person automatically thinks about heart attacks whenever she has unexpected chest pain; another worries incessantly about finances. This investment in the "anxious mind-set" can be evaluated using another cognitive therapy strategy called *cost–benefit analysis*. Worksheet 6.4 provides a self-help form for doing a cost–benefit analysis on your anxious thinking.

If you've been living with anxiety for a long time, your anxious way of seeing yourself and your world may have become an entrenched part of your life, and you may have forgotten the cost that it's exacting. Doing a cost–benefit analysis is a powerful way to increase your resolve to correct this faulty thinking. Reminding yourself of the heavy price you're paying for continuing to listen to your exaggerated thoughts and beliefs about threat and danger will help weaken your investment in "always assuming the worst."

> Use evidence gathering and a comprehensive cost–benefit analysis of your automatic anxious thoughts and beliefs as complementary interventions whenever you experience anxiety.

Self-Help Exercise 6.4: Do a Cost–Benefit Analysis

1. **Make extra copies of the form and then conduct a cost–benefit analysis by completing Worksheet 6.4 when you're not feeling anxious.** Write down a specific anxious thought or belief and then try to come up with immediate and longer-term advantages and disadvantages. Make sure you come up with specific pros and cons. Avoid general or vague reasons, which will not be helpful when you're anxious.

2. **Circle the advantages and disadvantages** that are most important to you.

3. Next try to **write down a more realistic, balanced thought or belief and then repeat the exercise for that thought.** You can refer back to the normalization card you completed in Step 1 for ideas about a more balanced, realistic way to think about your anxious concerns.

4. **Try to review the cost–benefit form immediately after anxiety episodes, spending several days on this exercise to correct, add, and delete various advantages/disadvantages to your thinking.** There may be some reasons that you overlooked when you completed the form when not feeling anxious.

5. **Review the cost–benefit form repeatedly while you're anxious** so you become so familiar with the disadvantages of anxious thinking that this comes to you automatically when you start to feel anxiety build.

One of the main worries for Jeremy, who had generalized anxiety, was *"I'm not saving enough money to protect myself from some future financial disaster."* Using the Cost–Benefit Analysis form, Jeremy recorded this worry as his anxious thought and then listed various advantages and disadvantages, circling those that were most important to him. For immediate and long-term advantages of the worry he listed:

1. It forced him to save more each month, and so his investments were slowly growing.

2. He watched his expenses much more closely.

3. He'd be better prepared to absorb a financial loss.

4. It ensured that he wouldn't lose the house or go bankrupt if he did lose his job.

5. He felt better about himself when he was saving.

Cost–Benefit Analysis

Date: _____

1. Briefly state the anxious thought or belief: _____

_____

Immediate and Long-Term Advantages	Immediate and Long-Term Disadvantages
1.	1.
2.	2.
3.	3.
4.	4.
5.	5.
6.	6.

Circle the costs and benefits that are most important to you.

2. Briefly state an alternative perspective: _____

_____

Immediate and Long-Term Advantages	Immediate and Long-Term Disadvantages
1.	1.
2.	2.
3.	3.
4.	4.
5.	5.
6.	6.

Circle the costs and benefits that are most important to you.

The disadvantages of the worry were:

1. The more he thought about not saving enough, the more anxious and tense he felt.

2. Once he started worrying about saving enough, he couldn't seem to stop; it consumed him.

3. He hadn't slept well because of worry over his investments.

4. There was little enjoyment in his life because he was constantly worried about finances.

5. He frequently deprived himself of little pleasures for fear of spending money.

6. He got into severe arguments with his wife over saving and spending money; she had threatened to leave.

7. He felt distant and uninvolved with his children because of his preoccupation with finances.

8. He spent long, frustrating hours each night monitoring his investments.

Although it took Jeremy considerable time to come up with a more balanced, realistic way to think about his finances, he eventually generated the following: *"I am saving enough money for temporary, moderate financial loss, but there is little I can do to guarantee protection against a sustained period of total financial ruin."* The advantages of this alternative perspective were:

1. Less anxiety about saving because he no longer needed to amass a huge safety net of savings.

2. More tolerance for stock market fluctuations.

3. Less need to monitor his investments.

4. More freedom to spend on everyday pleasures and comforts.

5. Fewer conflicts with his spouse over finances because of less attempt to control expenditures.

The possible disadvantages of the alternative perspective were:

> 1. He might end up with a smaller investment account because he was saving less money.
> 2. He would be prepared for a narrower range of future financial losses.

≳ Troubleshooting Tips ≲

You may not find cost–benefit analysis very helpful in reducing anxious thinking on its own. Often it's most helpful when used along with evidence gathering. Also, it's important not to treat cost–benefit analysis as an intellectual exercise but rather to deeply ponder and reflect on the disadvantages of exaggerating threat. It's important to feel these disadvantages emotionally, not just intellectually. To achieve this level of effect you must spend time with your cost–benefit form. You need to be adding to it, reviewing it frequently. You need to take it with you and read it over when experiencing anxiety. Remind yourself, "I can choose to think about the possibility of future threat, about the worst outcome, or I can choose to think about the less threatening alternative. Which way works best for me? Is my tendency to always focus on the worst possibility working well for me, or is it associated with a lot of negative effects? What's the cost of always assuming the worst, the most threatening or dangerous?"

Step 5: Decatastrophizing the Fear

Often our automatic thoughts and behaviors during anxiety episodes are attempts to avoid some imagined worst-case scenario or catastrophic outcome. Renee became intensely anxious whenever she felt congested, as if her airways were blocked. She would repeatedly clear her throat and try to take deep breaths. Although anxious about the possibility that she might suffocate, her ultimate fear was that the symptoms were due to a crippling degenerative neurological disease such as amyotrophic lateral sclerosis (ALS). She was so fearful of this disease that any mention of ALS caused an immediate anxiety response.

> To decatastrophize an imagined worst-case scenario that is the ultimate fear underlying excessive anxiety, you'll need to produce a detailed written elaboration of the catastrophe and practice repeated imaginal exposure to it and acceptance of a plan for coping with the disaster.

For many people suffering from anxiety, some imagined dreaded outcome has become a "nightmare" they seek to avoid at all costs. In such cases, confronting the imagined catastrophe is a powerful therapeutic tool for defusing its anxiety-inducing power. Does some ultimate catastrophe such as a terminal disease, fatal injury or accident, humiliating experience, recurrence of a past trauma, or some act of utter personal ruination underlie your anxiety? If so, decatastrophizing your imagined fear is an important cognitive therapy intervention for "deflating" anxious thinking.

Self-Help Exercise 6.5. Decatastrophizing the Fear

1. **Identify the worst-case scenario,** the ultimate fear that is the source of your anxiety. Decatastrophizing won't be effective unless you work with your deepest fear. Is it losing a loved one, contracting a deadly disease, being rejected by everyone and having to live a solitary life, failing miserably at an important life goal? Whatever the worst-case scenario or catastrophe, it must be the situation you dread most.

2. On a blank sheet of paper, **write down a detailed description of the worst-case scenario.** Describe in as much detail as you can what you imagine might happen to you. Why did this terrible tragedy happen? How has it affected you physically and emotionally? How have you responded to this imagined catastrophe? How have family, friends, your work colleagues responded? How do you imagine the catastrophe would affect your life; what might you still be able to do or no longer do? What's your imagined quality of life? How are you trying to cope?

3. Now spend some time **reviewing the catastrophe you wrote down.** Try to imagine what it would be like to live out this worst-case scenario. **Spend at least 30 minutes over several days** trying to imagine to the best of your ability what your life would be like living "in the eye of the storm," fully embracing the catastrophe. It's important not to simply read the catastrophic narrative like some intellectual exercise, but rather to get emotionally involved with the imagined scenario. After several days imagining your worst outcome, you will notice that the catastrophic image becomes much less anxiety provoking. When your anxiety has been reduced by half, it's time to go to the next step of decatastrophizing.

4. Work on developing **a problem-oriented coping plan** that you could use if the catastrophe ever struck. What would you do to minimize its effect? How would you get on with your work, family, social life, recreation, and leisure? How would you ensure at least some quality

of life? How could you encourage a more hopeful, optimistic attitude in this situation? Do you know anyone who had a similar catastrophe and yet coped well with adversity? Are there things they did that you could emulate? **Write down this coping plan on the same blank sheet of paper that you wrote your narrative.**

5. After writing down your coping plan, **each day for 2 weeks,** repeatedly imagine yourself coping effectively with the worst-case scenario. Continue with this exercise until you truly can imagine yourself dealing with the catastrophe and your anxiety over the catastrophe has reduced to no more than one-third of its original level.

Philip's catastrophic fear was failing to get into law school and having to live the rest of his life thinking of himself as "the family loser." In his story of what he imagined life would be like after being rejected from law school, he wrote about having to work in a menial low-paying job, never marrying or having a family, and never feeling like he could succeed. He repeatedly imagined this life scenario until his anxiety decreased by 50%. Then he imagined how he might cope with this imagined situation in a more effective manner—how he might find some meaning outside the legal profession, how he could interact with others and initiate close relationships without having "a big job," and how he could get the most out of life despite his disappointment. Philip thought about what it would be like if he had to resort to getting a job like one as an assistant manager at a video rental store. He wouldn't make much money, but having to share an apartment might mean he'd make a couple of close friends he could have fun with on weekends and evenings, and meanwhile he could work part-time on getting an MBA. This exercise drastically reduced Philip's fear of failure and his anxiety about law school admission.

> ⋛ Troubleshooting Tips ⋚
>
> If the decatastrophizing exercise doesn't help reduce your anxiety, make sure you're imagining a real catastrophe, the worst scenario you can imagine, no matter how unlikely, not just a fairly negative outcome. If you were anxious about the negative evaluation of your work colleagues, for example, you'd have to imagine something like having the entire office laugh at something ridiculous you said, not just the person in the next cubicle saying she wasn't sure she liked your new hairstyle as well as your

old one. The catastrophe you choose also has to be directly relevant to your anxious concern. Second, don't stop imagining the catastrophe the minute you feel anxious and don't just do the exposure once or twice, but numerous times. Finally, make sure the coping plan is realistic and really imagine doing this—you have to be able to get into the imagined coping plan for it to work.

Training yourself to become highly conscious of cognitive errors plays an important role in the process of learning to correct the thoughts and beliefs responsible for your anxiety.

Step 6: Correcting Thinking Errors

You've already done a lot of work on identifying particular cognitive errors entangled in your anxiety episodes. This strategy involves taking this ability "on the road" and identifying thinking errors whenever you become anxious.

Self–Help Exercise 6.6. Correcting Thinking Errors

1. Review what you wrote in Exercises 6.2 and 6.3 and write down any errors that are apparent in your anxious thinking.

2. **Then, over the next couple of weeks,** work on training yourself to become much more aware of your anxious thinking errors. Whenever you feel anxious, stop yourself and ask: "What am I thinking right now?" "Are there any errors or mistakes in how I'm thinking at this moment?" "Am I catastrophizing, jumping to conclusions, having tunnel vision or nearsightedness, emotional reasoning, or all-or-nothing thinking?" **On a blank sheet of paper,** write down some examples of common thinking errors that occurred during each anxiety episode. Within a few days you should have gathered many examples of anxious thinking errors. You can then be on the lookout for these errors whenever you feel anxious.

Philip noticed that the evidence he gathered for his anxious thought "I'm losing focus when I study; I don't understand anything" was loaded with numerous cognitive errors. *Tunnel vision* (he focused only on what he didn't know and ignored what he did understand), *emotional reasoning* (because he felt anxious, he assumed he must not be focusing), and *all-or-nothing think-ing* (if I can't remember everything when I study, then I must be losing my focus) were rampant when he became anxious about studying.

⋝ Troubleshooting Tips ⋜

If you need a reminder of all the various cognitive errors that can pop into your think-ing, review Table 3.2. If you still have trouble seeing the errors in your anxious thinking, start by picking out these errors in the thinking of your friends and family. Often it's easier to see the errors in other people's thinking. Once you've done this a few times, try becoming aware of your errors with nonanxious concerns, and then finally go back to identifying the errors during your anxiety episodes. You can ask a spouse or close friend who knows about your anxiety to help you identify the cognitive errors in your anxious thinking. Of course if you're in therapy, you'll be working on this skill during your sessions.

Step 7: Developing Alternative Perspectives

Based on what you've been reading, by now you are fully aware that your anxious thinking is exaggerated, excessive, and entirely unproductive, but you may be unsure of what a healthier view would look like. Or you might know of a healthier perspective but you can't seem to make yourself believe it when you feel anxious.

> It will take time and repeated practice before a healthier, more realistic interpretation or explanation of your anxious concern progresses from an intellectual view to an emotion-based conviction that you truly accept.

Before we get into issues of belief, let's focus on generating an alter-native, nonanxious perspective on your anxious concern. You can use Worksheet 6.5 to help you develop an alternative perspective.

Self-Help Exercise 6.7. Developing Alternative Perspectives

1. **Write down your automatic anxious or catastrophic interpretation, fol-lowed by your most desired or ideal outcome.** Then review the Gathering

Evidence form you previously completed (Worksheet 6.3) and **try writing out an interpretation or outcome that more closely matches the evidence that you recorded on that form. Finally, write down evidence for each of the three interpretations of your anxious concern.** Which of these three outcomes looks most believable based on the evidence? The following are some questions you can ask yourself when trying to generate an alternative explanation or interpretation.

- "Before I had problems with anxiety, how did I understand the anxious concern or interpret the situations that trigger the anxiety?"

- "How do other people who don't suffer from excessive anxiety think about the anxious concern or situation triggers of anxiety?"

- "Based solely on the evidence, what is the most likely interpretation or outcome of the anxiety-related situation?"

- "When I'm feeling calm and rational, what do I tend to think about the anxious concern or its triggers?"

2. After you've generated an alternative explanation for your anxious concern, try applying the more realistic explanation whenever you begin to feel anxious. **Continue to gather evidence from your daily experiences that the alternative explanation is the more realistic and accurate perspective.** Record this evidence on Worksheet 6.5.

Jody felt intensely anxious in public gatherings and so would avoid these situations as much as possible. Her automatic anxious thoughts when in a crowd were "I can't trust these people," "they are invading my personal space and pose a real threat to my sense of safety; therefore I must leave before I lose control." Jody's most desired interpretation or outcome was to never feel a sense of threat or mistrust when around unfamiliar people. However, based on the evidence and her recent experiences, she realized this was an unrealistic expectation. The more realistic alternative interpretation of her anxiety in public places was "I realize I will initially have feelings of unease and mistrust when in crowded places. I need to look around and focus my attention on the objective indicators that the present situation is safe and poses no personal threat. I need to remain steadfast and let the anxiety ebb and flow naturally. Even though my present anxiety is based on my past experiences of threatening crowds, that was then and this is now, and now I am presently in a shopping mall that poses the lowest level of actual personal threat and danger. My anxiety may be high, and I may even have a brief panic attack, but I can

Alternative Interpretations

Date: _____

1. Briefly state the catastrophic outcome (worst-case scenario) associated with your anxiety:

_____

_____

2. Briefly state the most desirable, ideal outcome (best possible scenario) associated with your anxiety:

_____

_____

3. Briefly state the most realistic (probable) outcome associated with your anxiety:

_____

_____

Evidence for the Dreaded Outcome (catastrophic view)	Evidence for the Ideal Outcome (most desired goal)	Evidence for the Most Probable Outcome (alternative view)
1.	1.	1.
2.	2.	2.
3.	3.	3.
4.	4.	4.

handle these feelings. My body is designed to handle these brief periods of intense anxiety and excitement."

⋛ Troubleshooting Tips ⋚

Discovering a more balanced, healthier perspective on your anxious concerns will take time and effort. If you have trouble thinking of an alternative view of your anxious concern, start by treating this as an "intellectual exercise." In other words, don't try to come up with a perspective you already believe or accept. Instead, try to distance yourself from the anxious concern. Imagine that the anxious concern or situation belonged to a friend or colleague. How would you advise that friend to think about her anxious concern? You could also ask close friends, a family member, or spouse how they see the situations that make you anxious. How do they think about anxiety itself? For example, when they get tense, feel chest discomfort, and have heart palpitations, how do they interpret these sensations in a nonanxious way? Adopt their nonanxious perspective as your alternative and work on gathering evidence for it so you eventually accept it over your anxious thinking. If you are in therapy, learning to accept an alternative perspective will be a major focus of your cognitive therapist.

Step 8: Practicing the Normalization Approach

Once you've done all the exercises in this chapter, you'll probably discover new insights into your anxious way of thinking. In light of the evidence you gather, the cost–benefit analysis, decatastrophizing, and generating alternatives, you can revisit what normal looks like.

Self–Help Exercise 6.8. Normalizing Anxiety

1. **Go back over the "normal anxiety card" you completed in Worksheet 6.1. Make some changes so this card reflects the most detailed and accurate alternative way to think about your anxious concern that you developed in the previous exercise.** Your normal anxiety card should address the following questions:

- ■ "What is the most probable outcome in this situation?"

- ■ "Is the most likely situation really that severe or intolerable?"

- ■ "How would I cope with the most likely outcome?"

- ■ "What aspects of this situation actually make it safer than I think?"

2. Refer to this new card every time you're anxious. **Continue to record any experiences that support this alternative explanation** as you did in the last self-help exercise. If you do this, within a couple of weeks you will become more and more invested in the alternative perspective and less convinced in your anxious thoughts of threat, danger, and vulnerability.

In light of the cognitive work completed in this chapter, Philip came up with the following alternative interpretation of the fear he experiences when he becomes so anxious that he can't study or retain any material:

> When I try to study for the LSAT, I do get quite anxious. However, only once or twice has the anxiety been so intense that I panicked. More often than not it's a queasy feeling in my stomach and some difficulty concentrating [*revised likelihood and severity estimates*]. I have found that the anxiety tends to ease if I take my time and focus on reading the study material rather than trying to quiz myself or memorize it. I actually do take in more material than I realize because when I go back over it I find that many of the concepts are familiar to me [*reduced helplessness*]. So I need to remember that anxiety does slow down my intellectual functioning and makes my studying less efficient. Therefore I need to practice the new study strategies that I learned that take into account that I'm studying under conditions of elevated anxiety [*reconsider safety aspects*].

CHAPTER SUMMARY

- ■ In cognitive therapy anxiety reduction occurs when we shift our automatic anxious way of thinking to a normalized perspective based on a more balanced, realistic view of threat, danger, and vulnerability.

- ■ Correcting exaggerated thoughts of threat and danger begins by recognizing one's ability to engage in a more normal thinking pattern during mild anxiety states.

- ■ Becoming skillful at catching automatic anxious thoughts and interpretations is a prerequisite to learning how to correct exaggerated thoughts of threat and danger.

- ■ Developing a "questioning" or skeptical attitude toward your initial anxious thought by diligently putting your anxious thinking to the test through evidence gathering is a key element in cognitive therapy.

■ Daily practice in questioning your anxious thinking is necessary for you to really begin to "feel doubtful" about your automatic anxious interpretations.

■ Repeatedly reminding yourself of specific short- and long-term costs of anxious thinking is another important cognitive strategy for strengthening doubt in the validity of your anxious mind.

■ Most people with anxiety have an underlying core fear that powers their anxiety state. Facing your worst-case scenario or ultimate fear and working through it with a reasonable and effective coping plan will help "defuse" the root cause of your anxiety.

■ Becoming more aware of the errors of thinking that occur during anxiety episodes is useful in evaluating the accuracy of automatic anxious thoughts and beliefs.

■ Developing a detailed, plausible, realistic, and probable alternative explanation or understanding of your anxious concern(s) and then using the "normalization card" to repeatedly apply this alternative perspective whenever you begin to feel anxious is the most important element in the radical transformation of your anxious mind.

7

Courageously Facing Fear

Webster's dictionary defines courage as "mental or moral strength to venture, persevere, and withstand danger, fear, or difficulty."[29] Based on this definition, we can see that courage is all around us. It takes courage to live and survive in this challenging and difficult society. Courage can be seen in how our neighbors, friends, family members, and colleagues face major life events and even in how they handle the minor, more mundane hassles of daily living.

You, too, act with strength and courage. The only difference between you and the people you consider courageous is that anxiety may make it difficult for you to recognize your own courage or to remember how well you've faced problems and challenges in the past. Anxiety may have become such a dominating force in your life that you now see yourself as weak, incompetent, and scared. The courage you once had seems inexplicably gone, replaced by a sense of resignation to cowardice. **The truth is, you still have courage. This chapter can help you rediscover your courage and use it in your work against anxiety.**

Even those whose acts of courage seem much more heroic than yours can suffer an apparent "loss of courage" and then reclaim it, as illustrated in the following story. Gerard, a 32-year-old 6'2" 220-pound combat soldier in top physical condition, had just returned from a second tour of southern Afghanistan, where he was frequently assigned foot patrols in dangerous villages, participated in convoys that came under enemy fire, and engaged in several firefights with the Taliban. Repeatedly he had placed himself in harm's way and on one occasion pulled an injured soldier to safety under intense fire. When he got home, however, Gerard's toughness and resilience seemed to desert him. Within a couple of months he had become so much more irritable, short-tempered, and anxious that his life started to crumble. He spent most days with a queasy feeling in his stomach and an overwhelming sense that something bad was about to happen. His anxiety seemed particularly intense around other people, so he started to avoid socializing. Crowds were particularly difficult, so he chose to stay at home alone. At the same time, his mood deteriorated and he felt depressed, uninterested, and hopeless about his current life and future. From a courageous, resilient soldier to a lonely, scared father cowering in his basement to avoid others—the fall could not have been more dramatic!

It took a few months of persuasion by his family for Gerard to agree that anxiety and depression had overtaken him and he needed help. At first he didn't realize that seeking help was itself a courageous thing to do, and it wasn't until he used a systematic program of behavioral change like the one we present in this chapter that he found he could face his anxiety with courage. You can too. Perhaps you've forgotten that you were once courageous, able to face the difficulties and uncertainties of life. But the good news is that you're still courageous, whether you recognize it or not. Anxiety cannot eliminate courage; it can camouflage it or override it, but it cannot eliminate it.

Acts of Courage

When was the last time you persevered at something or took a course of action that required strength, determination, and acceptance of some degree of risk? At first you may think you don't do anything that would fit with even the broadest definition of courage, but we find that's rarely the case. You may have had to confront someone about an issue you knew would be difficult, make a decision you knew would bring some hardship and uncertainty but was clearly the right decision, or face a difficult situation that was completely outside your control. Life has a way of presenting us with challenges we didn't invite, and that doesn't mean you haven't faced them with courage, whether it was moving to a city where you knew no one, starting a new job or school program, dealing with a serious illness, losing your job, having an intimate relationship end, parenting a difficult or rebellious child, or living with a partner who abuses drugs or alcohol.

To prove to yourself that you've demonstrated courage in the past, list on Worksheet 7.1 five or six past or current situations in which you displayed some degree of strength and courage. What were the situations, and what did you do that could be interpreted as an act of strength or courage?

Now look over your list and think about what you recorded. As you work through this chapter, keep Worksheet 7.1 close at hand as a reminder that you can act courageously. **Our goal is to help you tap into your enduring strength and to use that to face your anxiety courageously.**

> ⋛ **Troubleshooting Tips** ⋚
>
> If you feel uncomfortable writing down instances of your own courage, keep in mind that no one needs to see this list besides you. If you really can't think of yourself as ever having been courageous, try asking a close friend, partner, parent, or family member if he or she

Acts of Courage

Instructions: Briefly describe some fairly recent experiences that could be considered difficult and uncertain situations or circumstances in your life. Some of these may be major life events, such as loss of a loved one, or they could be minor, such as speaking up at a meeting when you were feeling especially anxious. In the second column, indicate what you did or how you coped with that situation in a way that indicates you displayed some perseverance, strength, and determination.

List of Difficult and Uncertain Life Circumstances, Situations, or Daily Demands	**Evidence of Strength and Courage** How did you cope with this situation that indicates you had strength, determination, and courage to overcome this situation?
1.	
2.	
3.	
4.	
5.	

can think of any experiences where you displayed strength of character and resourcefulness.

It's important to remind yourself of the strength and courage you've exhibited in everyday life challenges unrelated to your core fear and to realize you can use this resilience to courageously face your anxious concerns and overcome their debilitating effects.

Confronting Your Fears

When the anxious mind takes over, the automatic response is to escape or avoid the source of the anxiety. Gerard felt intense anxiety whenever he went shopping with his wife, so he stopped going with her. The trouble with escape and avoidance is that, while they may lead to an immediate reduction in anxious feelings and symptoms, they come at a high price. **Over the long term, escape and avoidance are powerful contributors to the persistence of your anxiety.** They reinforce your exaggerated thoughts of threat and danger and your belief that you're helpless to deal with the anxiety-provoking situation. Review your Anxiety Profile (Worksheet 5.9) to see how your anxious thinking in Part II and your thoughts of being helpless lead to avoidance and safety-seeking responses (Part III) to various anxiety-provoking situations (Part I).

In literally hundreds of research studies over the last 50 years, psychologists and psychiatrists have shown that the best antidote for fear and anxiety is repeated, systematic *exposure* to the feared situation.[5,30] Exposure can be defined as:

> *systematic, repeated, and prolonged presentation of external objects, situations, or stimuli, or internally generated thoughts, images, or memories, that are avoided because they provoke anxiety.*

Some examples of exposure might be repeatedly facing an unfamiliar situation that makes you anxious, acting more assertively or speaking up at a meeting, or traveling to new places. In other words, **exposure is mustering your courage and climbing out of your comfort zone.** There is no question that facing your fears through exposure takes determination, courage, and commitment. Yet time after time, with literally hundreds of anxious individuals, we have found that systematic, repeated, and prolonged exposure to their anxious triggers led to a rapid and sustained reduction in anxiety. Exposure can be thought of as a form of "desensitization" in which repeated exposure to fear triggers and the accompanying anxiety help you learn to see these situations more realistically and thus increase your tolerance for anxiety. For Gerard, exposure meant gradually and systematically increasing his contacts with other people, especially in public places like grocery stores, movie theaters, and shopping malls.

At first Gerard resisted the idea of exposure. Many people with anxiety try to ignore the "exposure message," and you may too. It's not easy to confront your fears, and you might be trying to persuade yourself right now that it doesn't even make sense to do so. If you noted on Worksheet 4.1 a pretty strong belief that facing your fears will only make things worse (item 1), you may find yourself also subscribing to a lot of the reasons for declining to expose yourself to anxiety triggers listed on Worksheet 7.2. Go through the checklist in Worksheet 7.2 and indicate which reasons make you hesitant to engage in an exposure program.

After completing the checklist, read over your reasons and ask yourself why you think this way about exposure. Are your reasons for not trying exposure based on something you've experienced or read? For example, if you checked the first reason, *"The anxiety will be too intense and I won't be able to stand it,"* is this based on a bad experience with previous therapy, on trying to do some exposure on your own and failing, or on something you read or were told? Or is it something that you're just worried about when it comes to exposure? Next, put this reason to the test. What's the evidence for and against the reason? Is this really a valid concern? Are there any cognitive errors or distortions in your thinking? Are you "catastrophizing" exposure, thinking it will be much worse than it really is? What would be an alternate, more balanced way to think about exposure? In Chapters 3–6 you've done a lot of work to learn to test your beliefs, and this is a perfect opportunity to call up that skill. If you can come up with even moderately effective challenges for your negative beliefs about exposure, you should be able to reach a point of willingness to try the exposure exercises in this chapter so that you can see for yourself that exposure will initially cause intense anxiety but that it will be bearable and that anxiety will decline naturally if left alone.

⌇ Troubleshooting Tips ⌇

If you're stuck on negative beliefs about exposure, particularly beliefs that it won't help, go back to Chapter 4 and remind yourself of Earl's mistakes that made his exposure exercises ineffective. Did you follow the seven "Rules for Success" in Chapter 4? If not, you may not have given yourself a fighting chance. Or perhaps your exposure exercises weren't well designed, also as defined in Chapter 4. Are you willing to give exposure another chance, this time making sure that you use well-designed exposure tasks? You also might reread how you filled out Worksheet 5.4 and some of the negative, upsetting thoughts you have when confronted with situations that trigger your anxiety. Maybe these thoughts are making it difficult to accept exposure to your fears. If so, use the cognitive skills you learned in Chapter 6 to challenge your negative thinking about facing the situations that trigger your anxiety.

Reasons Not to Do Exposure

Instructions: Read through this list of reasons why you might hesitate to engage in an exposure program and indicate whether each statement applies to you by checking "yes" or "no."

Reasons	Yes	No
1. The anxiety will be too intense and I won't be able to stand it.		
2. The anxiety will keep escalating and remain elevated for hours or even days on end.		
3. I've been feeling less anxious lately; exposure will only upset this relative calm.		
4. I have already exposed myself to fear situations, and it doesn't work; I still feel anxious.		
5. I need to reduce my anxiety to a manageable level before I start doing exposure.		
6. I need to learn better anxiety management strategies before I begin exposure.		
7. I've been anxious for so long that I don't see how exposure will help me.		
8. I just don't see how making myself more anxious will eventually cause me to feel less anxious.		
9. My anxiety is triggered by internal things like certain thoughts, images, memories, or worries. I don't see how exposure can help me.		
10. Exposure may be effective for others, but my anxiety is unique; I can't see how it could possibly help me.		
11. I am just too anxious now to engage in exposure. I'll wait until the medication "kicks in" before doing exposure.		
12. I don't have the courage, the "willpower" to do exposure.		

Misunderstandings about exposure should be questioned and evaluated just like any other belief about anxiety so that you can give yourself the best chance of success with systematic, repeated, and prolonged exposure to fear triggers—a highly effective therapeutic strategy for eliminating fear and anxiety.

The rest of this chapter is divided into two main tasks that make up the behavioral part of your self-help exercises for reducing anxiety: First you have to lay some groundwork to prepare and plan for exposure exercises. Then you actually have to go out into your daily routine and do the exercises. We'll walk you through the whole process. You will be working on the situational triggers of your anxiety (Part I) and the avoidance and safety-seeking responses (Part III) of your Anxiety Profile with the exposure exercises in this chapter, so keep Worksheet 5.9 handy. As with Chapter 6, however, we suggest you read Chapter 8 to help you plan both the cognitive and behavioral aspects of your mental fitness program before getting started on the exercises that follow.

Constructing an Effective Exposure Plan

Mary had intense social anxiety, and one of her exposure assignments involved calling a friend and inviting her to go to the movies. Mary put off doing the assignment until the day before her next therapy appointment. By this time the anticipatory anxiety had become so intense she was almost panicky. She eventually made the call, but the woman wasn't home. Mary tried to leave a message but in her anxiety forgot to leave her phone number. The friend never returned the call. Mary felt so much anticipatory anxiety and then relief when the woman wasn't home that she decided she would never again do another exposure exercise. Unfortunately, Mary was never able to work through this impasse with her therapist and so eventually quit treatment without achieving any progress with her social anxiety.

Mary, like Earl in Chapter 4, made probably the most common mistake that deters people from using exposure effectively: she dabbled in exposure and then felt much worse rather than better. Earl tried exposure once or twice, and only for a few minutes, and then decided it wasn't for him. These demoralizing experiences are why it's so important to spend time carefully constructing an exercise plan before beginning.

It's also important that you fully realize what to expect when you start an exposure treatment program. Don't expect it to be easy or painless! It will involve moderate to intense levels of anxiety, and you will want to "run." It will take courage and determination to face your fears and persist with the exposure tasks. You may want to turn back to the old habit of "run and hide." But if you persist—if you summon the courage you've shown in past situations—you will achieve significant success over your anxiety with exposure. However, you need to plan your exposure program, whether or not you are in therapy. We've already introduced a number of keys to an effective self-help exercise in Chapter 4. Building on those ideas, we introduce five more steps needed to construct an effective exposure plan:

1. Develop a written, systematic, step-by-step exposure plan that takes you through a hierarchy of anxiety triggers to address a particular core fear.

2. Identify and evaluate faulty thinking about exposure so you start unencumbered by doubt and harmful preconceived notions.

3. Plan to start with a moderate goal and work your way up gradually.

4. Commit to daily exposure practice.

5. Come up with a plan for coping with anxiety without resorting to false safety-seeking measures.

> A written exposure plan maximizes the effectiveness of this intervention and ensures that it does not make you more rather than less anxious.

Step 1: Develop an Exposure Plan

You begin your exposure plan by breaking down your fear triggers into a dozen or more graduated steps and then arranging these steps from least to most anxiety provoking.

> Make a list of all situations, objects, physical sensations, thoughts, or memories that trigger anything from mild to intense anxiety. Provide enough detail so you know what to do to elicit anxiety when you engage in exposure and rate the expected level of anxiety associated with each step.

You can start with the triggers you listed in Part I of your Anxiety Profile, but you will also need to review past worksheets (Worksheets 2.2 and 5.2) to develop your list of avoided situations. Probably each of these triggers was described in general terms, so you will need to break them down into more specific descriptions. For example, if your anxiety involved driving to unfamiliar places, your exposure plan would involve a series of tasks in which you gradually drive farther and farther away from home. It's important to generate at least 10 to 20 situations that range from mild to intense anxiety. Worksheet 7.3 is an Exposure Hierarchy form you can use to document your exposure plan. Make sure you include enough detail about what you must do in each situation to generate anxiety. **Remember, the goal of exposure to anxiety triggers is to make you feel anxious.** If you do an exercise without feeling anxious, the exposure will not be therapeutic. Also beside each exposure trigger, rate the situation from 0 to 100 on the amount of anxiety you expect to feel.

> Identifying exaggerated thoughts of threat and helplessness, critically evaluating them, and then replacing them with an alternative, more balanced perspective is an important therapeutic tool for managing your anxiety level during exposure.

Exposure Hierarchy

Date: _____

Instructions: On a blank sheet of paper, write down 15–20 situations, objects, physical sensations, or intrusive thoughts/images that are relevant to your anxious concerns. Select experiences that fall along the full range from those that trigger only slight anxiety and avoidance to experiences that elicit moderate and then severe anxiety and avoidance. Next rank-order these experiences from least to most anxious or avoidant and transfer the list into the second column on this form. In the first column, record the level of anxiety you expect with each entry, and in the second column describe the anxiety trigger that you try to avoid. In the third column, write down the core anxious thought associated with each situation if this is known to you.

	Expected Level of Anxiety/ Avoidance (0–100)	Briefly Describe the Anxious/ Avoided Situation, Object, Sensation, or Intrusive Thought/Image	Anxious Thinking What's so threatening, upsetting about this situation that makes you anxious or want to avoid it?
Least 1.			
2.			
3.			
4.			
5.			
6.			
7.			
8.			
9.			
10.			
11.			
12.			
13.			
14.			
Most 15.			

Reprinted with permission from *Cognitive Therapy of Anxiety Disorders* by David A. Clark and Aaron T. Beck (p. 268). Copyright 2010 by The Guilford Press.

Step 2: Target Anxious Thinking

Worksheet 7.3 also provides a column to record the anxious thoughts you may have during exposure to a particular trigger. It's important to be fully aware of the thoughts about threat, danger, and helplessness you may have during exposure and to critically confront this thinking before, during, and after you engage in exposure. You will recall from previous chapters that it's the thoughts that cause you to feel anxious in the situation. **Deal with the anxious thinking and you'll reduce your anxiety during exposure.**

Self-Help Exercise 7.1.
Creating Normalization Cards for Your Anxious Thoughts

This exercise is designed to help you think differently about the anxiety triggers you've been avoiding. Use the cognitive skills you learned in Chapter 6 (evidence gathering, cost–benefit analysis, decatastrophizing, etc.) to correct the anxious thoughts associated with each trigger in your exposure plan. Generate an alternative way of thinking about that anxiety trigger that is more balanced and less anxiety provoking. **Write down the alternative thinking on a "normalization card" or load it into your mobile device. If you have 15 triggers in your exposure plan, you should have 15 separate normalization cards.** These normalization cards will be similar to the one you completed in Chapter 6 (Self-Help Exercise 6.8) but will be specific to each situation you will tackle during exposure. The cards will be helpful for countering your anxious thinking when you do exposure to each situation.

Cynthia had suffered from intense social anxiety for many years. She developed a 20-step exposure plan that involved a range of social situations that elicited mild to intense anxiety. Here are her normalization cards for a mild, a moderate, and an intense anxiety trigger:

Situation: answering the telephone (10/100 anxiety rating).

Normalization card: When the phone rings, I feel slightly anxious because I don't know what to expect. It's okay to feel a little uneasy. I can say hello even when apprehensive, and I will quickly find out who is calling. If it's a friend, my anxiety will disappear rapidly; if it's a telemarketer, I can simply say "no thank you" and hang up immediately. If it's an important call like the doctor's office about an appointment, it's better to take it than to miss it.

Situation: attending a staff meeting at work (65/100 anxiety rating).

Normalization card: I'm going to feel quite anxious attending this staff meeting. I'll be thinking that everyone is staring at me and noticing that I'm uncomfortable. But is this really true? Look around at people. Are they really that interested in me? Do they have more important things to think about than me? I notice that some others in the room also look uncomfortable. Some look bored, and one or two people are falling asleep. It's probably more embarrassing to fall asleep. It's more likely that people are paying attention to more interesting things than me, like the person talking or the one falling asleep. I need to challenge this idea that I'm the center of attention with objective evidence.

Situation: speaking to her supervisor about a coworker who was treating her unfairly (95/100 anxiety rating).

Normalization card: I can expect to feel intense anxiety. This is not easy even for the most confident and assertive individual. However, I can't stand this situation at work any longer. Although I'll feel intense anxiety during the meeting with my supervisor, in the end I'll experience less stress at work if we can deal with this problem. I'm going to write down the main points I want to make with the supervisor. I'm going to admit to her that I feel very uncomfortable complaining about a coworker, and then I'll tell her exactly what has happened and how it has affected me. Even though I'm feeling anxious, I can refer to my notes and I'll be able to tell whether or not the supervisor understands my complaint by how she responds. Most people would feel apprehensive in this situation, but they just get on with it and do it. I can do the same.

Step 3: Plan to Start Moderately and Resolve to *Pace Yourself*

It's important to do exposure in a graduated fashion, starting your exposure somewhere in the middle of the hierarchy in Worksheet 7.3, where you experience moderate anxiety. If you start too low in the hierarchy, you waste a lot of time doing things that cause only mild anxiety. If you start too high, you'll feel overwhelmed with intense anxiety. **Remember, the goal of exposure is to generate moderate anxiety so you can experience the anxiety decreasing over time with repeated practice. In the process you learn that the situation is not dangerous and you're not helpless.**

Also be sure to stick with one task and do it over and over until you can do it with only slight feelings of anxiety. Each time you do exposure you should have ready access to your normalization card and challenge any thoughts of exaggerated threat and helplessness. Cynthia, for example, started her exposure with "attending staff

> Exposure is like running a marathon: pacing is everything! If you start with a task that provokes moderate anxiety and still find the exposure too overwhelming, drop back to a less intense task and work on it. If the exposure is too easy, proceed up the hierarchy until you do a task that is moderately challenging.

meetings" because this caused her moderate anxiety. She decided to go to as many staff meetings as possible and gradually moved herself closer to a prominent seat in the room. Carl had intense fear of making mistakes and so engaged in repeated reassurance seeking. He started his exposure with confronting his doubts about whether his reports were perfectly accurate and well written. Joan had panic attacks and so avoided crowds or public places. Her exposure began with entering a moderately sized clothing store where only a few people would be present.

Step 4: Commit to Practice, Practice, and More Practice

Successful exposure is like physical exercise: practice is critical! The more exposure you do, the better the outcome. You should aim to do some exposure every day, especially at the beginning. Also make sure you do at least 30 minutes of exposure each time. The number-one reason that exposure treatment fails in anxiety is that people do too little exposure. The problem with brief and occasional exposure is it can have a reverse effect. **Occasional or brief exposures can actually INTENSIFY your anxiety.** You are more likely to feel overwhelmed with brief exposure (5 to 15 minutes). It will reinforce your faulty anxious beliefs that the situation is highly threatening and that you are helpless to deal with your anxiety. You'll end up discounting what you've written on your normalization card and conclude that the best strategy is to return to avoiding the situation.

Darren had an intense fear of crossing bridges. He had done a number of exposures dealing with bridges and now was confronting an exposure task that involved severe anxiety. One of us (D.A.C.) accompanied Darren to a bridge, and we planned to step on the bridge sidewalk. Darren's anxiety escalated rapidly as we walked toward the bridge. However, every few feet we stopped and waited for his anxiety to drop to a level that he felt was manageable. We then proceeded a few more feet, stopped, and let the anxiety settle. At the same time, Darren challenged his anxious thinking about the danger in what he was doing and that his anxiety was intolerable. Finally we reached the bridge, the whole exercise taking 45 to 60 minutes. We waited there for quite a while until Darren felt the anxiety decline significantly. This exposure proved pivotal in Darren's therapy because it provided objec-

> The success of exposure depends on its "dosage." Do the same exposure task over and over for at least 30 minutes until you can do the task with only slight feelings of apprehension.

tive evidence that he could face bridges. From this point forward, Darren began driving across bridges and within 2 weeks was reporting minimal anxiety.

Step 5: Develop a Coping Strategy

The whole point of exposure is to generate anxiety and then let it decline naturally. So you will be anxious during exposure. Having a list of coping strategies that you can call on will help you get through it. The goal is to ensure that you remain in the exposure situation without engaging in escape or a safety behavior that would interfere with the natural decline in anxiety. The following are some constructive coping strategies you can use to deal with anxiety and sustain exposure to the anxious situation.

1. **Modify anxious thinking.** Write down any anxious thoughts experienced during exposure, evaluate them as you learned to do in Chapter 6, and substitute more balanced, realistic alternative thinking. *Remember, modifying your thoughts of danger and helplessness will lower your anxiety level.*

2. **Focus on physical symptoms.** Focus all your concentration on specific physical symptoms of anxiety, such as feelings of muscle tension, heart palpitations, nausea, or breathlessness. Rather than deny these symptoms, accept them, embrace them, and practice experiencing them as normal heightened physical arousal.

3. **Find evidence of safety.** Consciously and deliberately look around your exposure environment and pick out evidence that the environment is safe. How are other people reacting in this situation? What characteristics of the situation indicate that it is safe, not dangerous?

4. **Control your breathing.** Some people find it helpful to focus on their breathing when anxious. Maintain a breathing rate of 8–12 breaths per minute. Make sure you don't overbreathe (hyperventilate) or take shallow breaths.

5. **Initiate relaxation.** Some people find physical relaxation or meditation calming when anxious. Others, however, find that trying to relax physically when anxious is frustrating and ineffective. *You can try out this coping strategy, but never use it to avoid feeling anxious.*

6. **Visualize mastery.** You can visualize yourself slowly and successfully mastering the exposure task either before you enter the situation or just after you begin. Imagining yourself successfully doing the exposure can boost your confidence and positive expectations about the task.

7. **Increase physical activity.** Some people find it helpful to be physically active during exposure. Rather than stand or sit, you could walk around in the exposure situation to help channel some of the physical arousal you feel. *Never use physical activity to avoid anxiety or the exposure task.*

If for some reason a particular coping strategy dramatically reduces your anxiety level, stop using it. That's a good sign that you're using it to escape anxiety or to seek safety. Remember, the whole point of exposure is to let the anxiety decline naturally. We'll tell you more about how to avoid safety seeking later in the chapter.

Develop a list of coping strategies you can use to help you remain in the exposure situation until anxiety has declined naturally, but remember that the purpose of coping is to make anxiety more tolerable and not to eliminate it entirely.

Doing Exposure

Now that you've developed a detailed exposure plan, it's time to put it into action. Worksheet 7.4 is a form you can use to record your exposure practice sessions. **Before you begin, you may want to review all the steps in your exposure plan. If you're working with a therapist, discuss the plan with her and agree on how to conduct your exposure assignments. If you're not engaged in therapy, discuss the plan with a close friend or family member. Does she think the plan looks systematic and reasonable? Make adjustments to gaps in your plan or realign the steps if they don't progress in a logical manner.**

Table 7.1 illustrates Gerard's exposure plan for dealing with his fear and avoidance of crowded public places. Notice the graded nature of the exposure plan. Gerard started with "going to the grocery store with my wife," since that situation caused him a moderate level of anxiety. His most prominent anxious thoughts were "I'll lose control and experience intense anxiety," "People will notice there is something wrong with me and wonder if I'm going berserk," and "I'll have flashbacks to the crowded marketplaces in Afghanistan." Gerard noticed that his anxiety escalated when he started thinking like this, and he tended to bolt from the situation, convinced he needed to escape before the anxiety became unbearable. So it was important that Gerard stay focused on his normalization card ("I am still in control even though I feel anxious; no one is looking at me or even interested in me; even if I'm thinking about Afghanistan, it doesn't change the reality that I'm safely back home in a grocery store"), ground himself in the present moment of being in the grocery store, and allow the anxiety to dissipate naturally through continued exposure.

Self-Help Exercise 7.2. Practicing Exposure

Begin practicing exposure on a daily basis by starting with a moderately anxious situation from your exposure plan. Use the Exposure Practice form

Exposure Practice

Date: _____

Instructions: Keep a record of your daily exposure practice sessions using this form. Be sure to record the initial, middle, and final anxiety rating as well as the type of exposure task completed and its duration.

Date and Time	Exposure Task	Duration (minutes)	Initial Anxiety (0–100)	Midpoint Anxiety (0–100)	Endpoint Anxiety (0–100)

TABLE 7.1. **Gerard's Exposure Plan for Fear and Avoidance of Public Places**

Rank (least to most)	Exposure task	Anxiety rating (0–100)
1.	Answering the telephone	15
2.	Going to the corner store for a quart of milk	20
3.	Waiting in line at the bank	35
4.	Going grocery shopping with my wife	45
5.	Going grocery shopping alone	65
6.	Walking around a crowded mall alone while my wife shops	70
7.	Eating at a table against the wall at a waitered restaurant	75
8.	Eating at a table in the middle of the room in a waitered restaurant	85
9.	Going to a house party and not able to leave for 2 hours	85
10.	Attending a sold-out movie and having to sit in the middle of the row	90
11.	Eating in the food court at the mall on a busy Saturday afternoon	93
12.	Shopping at Walmart on a busy Saturday afternoon, pushing a shopping cart around the busiest aisles	95

(Worksheet 7.4) to record the outcome of each exposure practice session. You should complete Worksheet 7.4 while you are doing the exposure exercise so you get an accurate picture of changes in your anxiety. If you're working with a therapist, review your practice form at the beginning of each therapy session. Otherwise, show a trusted friend or family member your practice form so there is someone who can hold you accountable for sticking with your exposure plan.

If you have done a particular exposure task three or four times, and each time your anxiety declined by half when you finished the task (e.g., dropped from an initial level of 80/100 to 40/100), then you've been successful and are ready to move on to the next task in your exposure hierarchy (Worksheet 7.3). If your anxiety does not decline after three or four attempts or even escalates, return to an easier task in your exposure hierarchy. Practice that task again until you're ready to return to the more difficult exposure task.

> ⋛ **Troubleshooting Tips** ⋚
>
> In their 1985 treatment manual for cognitive therapy of anxiety disorders, Beck and Emery[4] proposed a five-step *AWARE* strategy to deal with anxiety. This strategy is particularly helpful for coping with the elevated levels of anxiety that occur during exposure.
>
> 1. **A**ccept anxiety. Instead of fighting against anxiety, agree to receive it; welcome it as part of the exposure experience.
>
> 2. **W**atch your anxiety. Observe the symptoms of anxiety in a nonjudgmental manner. Rate your anxious experience and then watch it ebb and flow. Separate yourself from the anxiety and observe it like you were standing on the sidelines and watching a parade march by.
>
> 3. **A**ct with the anxiety. Normalize the exposure situation and act *as if* you were not anxious. Slow yourself down if necessary, take a couple of good breaths, and stay connected to the situation.
>
> 4. **R**epeat the steps. Repeat Steps 1–3 until your anxiety decreases to a milder, more acceptable level.
>
> 5. **E**xpect the best. Don't be surprised by anxiety. Learn to expect that you will experience anxiety in exposure situations. Correct any false expectations that anxiety can be utterly defeated for all time. Instead replace this with the goal of strengthening your ability to tolerate anxiety. *In this way you take control of anxiety rather than letting it control you.*

Don't procrastinate—start your exposure program today! Most people with anxiety find the anticipation more anxiety-provoking than the actual task. It will probably be less difficult than you expect.

"Supercharge" Your Exposure Exercises

One of the best ways to make your exposure exercises even more powerful for reducing anxiety is to turn them into what cognitive therapists call behavioral experiments. *Behavioral experiments* are:

structured, planned tasks designed to collect evidence for and against an anxious belief about threat or danger and personal vulnerability.

We believe behavioral experiments are an especially effective way to enhance exposure because exposure therapy is thought to work by correcting maladaptive fear beliefs and help the person relearn that fearful situations are actually safe.[30] So why not tailor your exposure exercises so they more directly target anxious thinking and beliefs?

In cognitive therapy for anxiety disorders, behavioral experiments combine the evidence-gathering skills you learned in Chapter 6 with the exposure-based exercises discussed in this chapter. It's a great way to deal with negative expectations and other anxious thoughts that could prevent you from doing exposure. For example, Gerard believed he would become overwhelmed with anxiety and lose control if he ventured into a crowded grocery store. After generating evidence for and against this belief, Gerard's therapist noted that the best way to evaluate this belief would be to go into a crowded grocery store, stay there for at least 30 minutes, and record what happened to his anxiety. Would his anxiety become overwhelming, and would he lose control? Gerard agreed to the exposure assignment and to record how he made out doing the assignment. He experienced high levels of anxiety, which gradually declined to the mild/moderate level after 30 minutes. He discovered that the anxiety did not become overwhelming and that he didn't lose control. He also made a bonus observation: no one seemed to notice him or could detect what he was feeling inside. This experience provided Gerard with evidence that his exaggerated thoughts about the probability and severity of threat and helplessness ("I'll have overwhelming anxiety and lose control") were not supported by real-life experiences. Gerard was then able to use this experience to counter future anxious thoughts about being overwhelmed and out of control (e.g., "I remember that when I went to the crowded grocery store last month I didn't become overwhelmed with anxiety and loss of control. Clearly, then, these fears are false and not supported by reality").

Worksheet 7.5 is a form that you can use along with the Exposure Practice form (Worksheet 7.4) when doing exposure exercises.

Self–Help Exercise 7.3.
Supercharging Your Exposure Exercises

Before engaging in the exposure task, write down on Worksheet 7.5 what you think is the most threatening possible outcome of doing the exposure exercise. Then write down what you think is the most probable, realistic outcome, and finally write down how you expect to benefit from doing the exposure exercise. After completing the exposure assignment, which you recorded on Worksheet 7.4, turn to Worksheet 7.5 and write a brief description of the exposure exercise, what you actually did during exposure, and its outcome. Did the exposure go much better or worse than you expected?

Behavioral Experiment Record

Date: _____

1. What is most threatening, the worst outcome that could happen from doing this exposure task? _____

2. What is a more realistic likely outcome from doing this exposure task? _____

3. What are the positive effects, the benefits you expect from doing this exposure task? _____

Description of Exposure Task	What Did You Think, Feel, and Do during the Exposure Task?	The Outcome—What Actually Happened

One of the best ways to improve the anxiety-reducing potential of exposure is to use it to conduct a behavioral test of your anxious thoughts and beliefs—an opportunity to collect evidence that contradicts those faulty thoughts of threat and helplessness that form the core fear in your anxiety.

⋛ Troubleshooting Tips ⋜

Exposure is hard work, and it's easy to get discouraged. If you're tempted to conclude that exposure is not for you, keep in mind that numerous research studies have shown that exposure is probably the most effective and quickest remedy for anxiety.[5,30,31] In the following list of reasons that an exposure program might fail, circle the experiences you had in recent exposure exercises.

Anxiety did not decrease during the exposure session.

Had one of my worst panic attacks while doing the exposure task.

Terminated exposure just a few minutes after starting it.

Was overwhelmed with anticipatory anxiety.

Could do the exposure task only if accompanied by friend or family.

Took an antianxiety medication before doing the exposure task.

Did only a small part of the exposure exercise.

Tried hard to remain calm and relaxed during exposure but failed.

Did not experience any anxiety at the end of the exposure task.

Experienced heightened anxiety several hours after completing the exposure task.

Became convinced that the exposure exercise was too difficult and could stress me out too much.

Felt discouraged and defeated after doing the exposure exercise.

Tried to distract myself as much as possible during exposure.

Avoided any reminders of the exposure situation between exposure sessions.

Reviewing the items you circled, how can you ensure the same mistakes do not happen again? Write out some changes you can make in your exposure plan to ensure that it's more successful.

Carol had an intense fear of getting sick and would repeatedly check in the mirror to see if she looked flushed or ask her coworkers whether they thought she looked unwell. Carol's core fear (catastrophe) was that she would get sick and start vomiting. Carol set up an exposure plan with her therapist that involved her wearing a sweater at work, which would make her feel hot, somewhat flushed, and uncomfortable. She was to refrain from checking her complexion in the mirror or asking coworkers whether she appeared ill. The following week she reported to her therapist how discouraged she was about her attempts at exposure. She had tried wearing the sweater, but after 20 minutes of feeling hot she became intensely anxious, thinking that maybe this could cause her to become sick, and so she removed the sweater. She made a couple of other attempts at wearing the sweater to work later in the week but gave up because the whole exercise was stressing her out.

Carol and her cognitive therapist decided she should drop down to a task with a lower anxiety rating. Her therapist emphasized that in her case it was important to undergo sustained (45- to 90-minute) daily exposure to what she feared. They also discovered that Carol was still very intolerant of anxiety and had a number of faulty beliefs about exposure ("What if I get hot and flushed, which actually causes me to get sick?"; "What if I become so anxious I have a panic attack at work?"; "What if my anxiety remains unbearably elevated for several days after exposure?"). Carol and her therapist evaluated these beliefs and strengthened her normalization card so she could deal with the anxious thoughts that undermined her exposure efforts.

If you're not having success with exposure, examine the reasons you circled in the preceding list:

- Do you need to drop down to a less anxiety-provoking task? If you tried the full duration of exposure and just couldn't tolerate the intense anxiety, you may have picked a task that's too intense.

- Do you need more prolonged and frequent exposure? Most cases of failed exposure are caused by individuals doing only brief exposure once or twice a week.

- Are you trying to do the exposure without feeling anxious? This is entirely unrealistic and actually defeats the purpose of exposure. You're supposed to feel anxious and learn to let the anxiety decline naturally. So you should stop all efforts to make yourself feel less anxious and instead fully engage yourself in the exposure task.

- Were you overwhelmed by anxious thinking during exposure? Again write down your anxious thoughts, evaluate them, and correct them with more realistic alternative thinking. Turn your exposure into "behavioral experiments" and use Worksheet 7.5 to correct negative expectations and other anxious thoughts that may undermine your efforts to do exposure.

Reducing Reliance on Safety

It takes courage to engage in exposure to your fears. Identify your problems with exposure, revise your exposure plan, and then return to your daily practice sessions.

It's always important to be aware of any thoughts or behaviors that you engaged in during exposure that are attempts to reduce or eliminate anxiety. Like escape and avoidance, safety seeking is an attempt to reduce anxiety, but these anxiety-control strategies are "false" because they don't actually protect us from danger.[15] Instead, they are unhelpful coping responses that ultimately strengthen anxiety because they reinforce the anxious mind's exaggerated thoughts of threat and helplessness. Use Worksheet 7.6 to record any false coping strategies you used during exposure that may have undermined its effectiveness. Look back at the third section of your Anxiety Profile (Worksheet 5.9) to remind yourself of the safety-seeking and coping strategies you should target for change.

Gerard was able to identify a number of false safety-seeking responses when he began his exposure to public places. At first he was terrified of losing control and feeling intense anxiety. So he took an Ativan before doing the exposure task. He also did not let his wife leave his side when they went shopping, and he tried to distract himself by thinking about pleasant activities. He kept telling himself that "everything will be all right," that he needed to try hard to suppress his anxiousness so that he wouldn't lose control, and to "just calm down." Gerard learned that these responses only escalated the anxiety and sense of being out of control during exposure. After identifying his "false safety-seeking" responses, Gerard worked hard to refrain from engaging in these strategies during subsequent exposure sessions. He eventually left his medication at home, let his wife go off shopping so he was left in the mall by himself for longer periods of time, kept himself focused on feelings of anxiety rather than trying to distract himself with pleasant thoughts, and stopped trying to calm himself down.

To maximize the effectiveness of exposure, refrain from all efforts to control or eliminate anxiety. Identify your false safety-seeking responses and work on eliminating them from your exposure exercises.

This resulted in a significant improvement in the effectiveness of exposure, so that in a couple of weeks Gerard was spending considerable time in crowded stores and malls without feeling overwhelmed with anxiety.

⋛ Troubleshooting Tips ⋚

Eliminating safety seeking can be difficult because you've probably used these strategies for years to reduce anxiety. If your initial efforts are unsuccessful, try weaning yourself off the safety response more gradually. Gerard, for example, at first couldn't leave his medication at home, so he left it in the car while doing exposure to crowded stores and then eventually left it at home. Also make sure you don't substitute one safety-seeking response for

Exposure Safety Seeking

Instructions: Use this form to record any thoughts or behaviors used during exposure to control or reduce anxiety. After identifying unhelpful coping responses, write in the last column what you can do to ensure that you don't fall back on false safety-seeking responses when repeating this exposure task. [Review your responses to Part III of your Anxiety Profile (Worksheet 5.9) to help with completing this form.]

Exposure Task	False Safety Behavior	False Safety Thoughts	How I'll Reduce Safety Seeking
1.			
2.			
3.			
4.			
5.			

another. Carol stopped asking people whether she looked well (a safety-seeking response) but then started looking up symptoms on the Internet (another safety-seeking response). The main point is that anything that dramatically reduces or eliminates anxiety will undermine the effectiveness of exposure.

CHAPTER SUMMARY

▪ Courage is an important element in overcoming fear and anxiety. We've all had times in life when we've courageously confronted very difficult life situations. It is now time to harness that internal strength and resolve to overcome your anxious concern.

▪ Exposure is a highly effective psychological treatment for anxiety. However, many people with anxiety refuse to engage in systematic exposure to their anxiety triggers because of faulty and exaggerated beliefs about fear exposure. It's important to identify, evaluate, and restructure these beliefs before giving up on exposure therapy.

▪ It's important to have a well-developed plan before starting exposure. This should include a written hierarchy of anxiety triggers ranging from least to most anxiety provoking. Exposure should take a systematic, graduated approach with daily, prolonged exposure sessions. You should identify and evaluate any anxious thinking that might undermine the effectiveness of exposure and develop a "normalization card" that will remind you of healthy coping strategies while engaged in an exposure task.

▪ Use the *AWARE* strategy to cope with your anxiety, especially during exposure tasks.

▪ The benefits of exposure can be maximized by turning your exercises into behavioral experiments that correct anxious thoughts and negative expectations about exposing yourself to anxiety.

▪ If exposure does not lead to a significant reduction in anxiety, it's important to troubleshoot your exposure plan. Identify what went wrong during your exposure assignments, make the necessary adjustments, and resume your schedule of daily exposure sessions.

▪ False anxiety management or safety-seeking behaviors can undermine the effectiveness of exposure and intensify anxiety. It's important to wean yourself off all cognitive and behavioral safety-seeking responses (attempts to control anxiety) and replace them with a more adaptive approach to anxiety.

8

Let's Talk Strategy

You've started a new venture, a cognitive way to tackle your problem with anxiety. As with all ventures, you need a plan—a road map that guides you in applying the skills learned in the first seven chapters to your unique experience of anxiety. You may have heard this Normal Vincent Peale quote: "Plan your work, work your plan. Lack of system produces that 'I'm swamped' feeling." Nothing could be truer when it comes to working on anxiety. In this workbook you've been introduced to the cognitive therapy approach and to various strategies you can use to overcome anxiety. If you tried some of the exercises in Chapters 6 and 7 and ended up feeling a bit overwhelmed by where to go with them, you now know why we suggested formulating a plan in this chapter before really starting work on the exercises. In this chapter we'll show you how to develop your own cognitive therapy plan, provide an illustration of an intervention plan, and then discuss whether you should consider reading one or all of the specialized chapters that follow.

Developing a cognitive therapy plan for tackling your anxiety problems will keep you focused, effective, and committed to working on your anxiety.

Why You Need a Plan

1. **Maintains goal direction.** In Chapter 1 (Worksheet 1.2) you wrote down some goals you wanted to achieve from doing this workbook. Having a treatment plan will help ensure that you're working toward those goals.

2. **Keeps you focused.** You completed your Anxiety Profile in Chapter 5 (Worksheet 5.9). It's important to apply the cognitive and behavioral skills you learned in Chapters 6 and 7 to the various elements of your anxiety profile. Having a treatment plan will help you do this.

3. **Promotes a systematic, organized approach.** Cognitive therapy works best when you break your anxiety down into its components (as you did in your

Anxiety Profile) and then work on each component in a systematic way. A treatment plan will help you work on your anxiety in a more organized manner to maximize its effectiveness.

4. **Sustains commitment.** Athletes training for a competition always plan out their training routine and schedule. They know this is critical to getting the most out of their physical training. The same holds true for "mental fitness training." A cognitive therapy plan for improving your "mental fitness for anxiety" will help you maintain a disciplined approach to working on your anxiety.

5. **Enables evaluation.** It's important to discover the strategies in Chapters 6 and 7 that work best for you and the ones that are less helpful. Structuring your cognitive therapy work around a plan based on your anxiety profile will help you evaluate progress and identify the parts of your anxiety problem that need more work.

The Anxiety Work Plan

Use Worksheet 8.1 to develop your Anxiety Work Plan. You should have your Anxiety Profile (Worksheet 5.9) handy, as well as the other worksheets you completed so you can refer to them as you develop your work plan. Notice that the work plan is divided into three parts that correspond to your anxiety profile—situations and other triggers of anxiety, the evaluation of threat (automatic anxious thinking), and coping responses (attempts to control or reduce anxiety). **You should select one target from each section—a trigger, an anxious thought, and a coping response—and work on these three targets simultaneously. Once you've made progress on these symptoms, move on to the next set of three symptoms.**

Anabel felt anxious taking any public transport, especially the subway. In her work plan she started with just going to a subway station and watching the trains go by (situation trigger), correcting the threatening thought "What if I have a panic attack in the station?" and preventing herself from leaving at the first sign of anxiety (escape coping response). After successfully reducing her anxiety in the subway station, Anabel moved on to the next phase in her work plan, which involved taking a subway ride with a friend in a nearly empty car.

To complete your Anxiety Work Plan, take the following steps. **You will need to make multiple copies of Worksheet 8.1, because you will have more than 10 entries on your work plan.**

Step 1: Target Anxiety Symptoms

Begin by completing the first column in all three parts of Worksheet 8.1. Write out the specific characteristics of your anxiety in each cell of the column by referring to what

Anxiety Work Plan

Instructions: Complete the first three columns as a planning exercise before you start working on your anxiety. When you have finished working on a particular anxiety symptom, record whether you found the intervention effective in the final column.

Targeted Anxiety Symptom	Intervention Exercises	Self-Help Schedule	Outcome
PART I. ANXIETY TRIGGERS (situations, etc.)			
1.			
2.			
3.			

(*cont.*)

Targeted Anxiety Symptom	Intervention Exercises	Self-Help Schedule	Outcome
PART II. THREAT EVALUATION (anxious thinking)			
4.			
5.			
6.			

(*cont.*)

Targeted Anxiety Symptom	Intervention Exercises	Self-Help Schedule	Outcome
PART III. COPING RESPONSES (avoidance, safety seeking, etc.)			
7.			
8.			
9.			
10.			

you recorded on your Anxiety Profile. First write down all the situations, thoughts, physical sensations, that you recorded as anxiety triggers in Part I of the Anxiety Profile. Each trigger should be written in a separate cell. For example, if you listed five situational triggers for your anxiety (e.g., meeting unfamiliar people, taking an elevator, feeling warm and hot, thinking about finances, speaking up at a meeting), you would have five different entries in the first column of Part I. Then move on to Part II and in the same column list any physical sensations that you find particularly upsetting, even frightening (e.g., heart palpitations, difficulty breathing). This will be found on the "evaluation of physical sensations" line of Part II in the Anxiety Profile.

It's critical that you also list in Part II of the plan the main automatic thoughts about threat, danger, worst outcomes, or catastrophe that come to your mind when you're anxious. You will probably have three or four main anxious thoughts, so each one should be recorded in a separate cell. For example, you would have three separate entries in column 1 if your automatic anxious thoughts were "What if people notice that I'm anxious and think I must be mentally ill?" and "What if this chest pain really is a heart attack?" and "What if my child gets seriously injured while with the babysitter?" Next write down all the typical cognitive errors (tunnel vision, all-or-nothing thinking, overgeneralization, etc.) you tend to make when feeling anxious. These can all be written in one cell because you will want to work on all the errors at the same time. You should also write down any faulty beliefs you may have about anxiety from the last entry in Part II of your Anxiety Profile. Again each belief, such as "I can't let myself get anxious because it could develop into a panic attack" or "If I don't get control over worry, it could drive me crazy," should be recorded in a separate cell.

In Part III of the plan, write down from your Anxiety Profile all the different ways you attempt to cope with anxiety. Again record separately each thought about helplessness, any additional things you avoid not already covered by the situational triggers, safety-seeking responses, other anxiety control strategies, and any worries you have about anxiety or other issues in your life. Overall it is very likely that you will end up with 15 to 20 different anxiety symptoms that you will want to target in your Anxiety Work Plan.

> Breaking down your anxiety into individual symptoms—specific anxiety triggers, anxious thoughts about threat and danger, and coping responses—is an essential step because it enables you to target exactly what needs to be changed to reduce anxiety.

Step 2: List Intervention Exercises

In the second column, write down some specific interventions from Chapters 6 and 7 that you can use to work on each anxiety symptom described in the first column. There will be two, maybe three, exercises that you'll want to use for each symptom. Some of the exercises, like evidence gathering and exposure, will be useful for many of the symptoms you listed in column 1, so don't worry if you find yourself writing in the same intervention exercise for multiple symptom targets. Because of space limitations, write down on Worksheet 8.1 the section headings, self-help exercise numbers, and page number of the various interventions you will use for the targeted symptom. You will also need to review the worksheets in Chapters 6 and 7 to decide how you will carry out the intervention for each symptom.

Hannah was anxious about her friendships and whether people really liked her. Her anxiety was often triggered by a social event, such as having lunch with friends. She would worry afterward that she might have said something that offended her friends. Hannah wrote on her Anxiety Work Plan that one of her anxiety triggers was "having lunch with a close friend." In Part II the physical sensation recorded in column 1 was a nauseated feeling in the stomach, which she interpreted as "I must have said something wrong." Her automatic anxious thought was "I've offended my friend, and now she won't like me." For her coping responses in Part III, Hannah wrote that her helplessness thoughts were "I'm so stupid and careless in my conversation" and her main coping response was worry—she would rehash over and over in her mind the conversation with her friend and whether she might have said something rude or offensive.

For interventions to tackle the situational triggers of her anxiety Hannah wrote in the second column that she would develop an exposure plan, a normalization card for use during social interactions, and a list of potential coping strategies and actually schedule regular social engagements with friends (Self-Help Exercises 7.1 and 7.2). However, for her core anxious thought "I've offended my friend, and she won't like me" and helplessness thought "I'm so stupid and careless in my conversation," she decided that gathering evidence (Exercise 6.3), correcting thinking errors (Exercise 6.6), decatastrophizing (Exercise 6.5), and developing an alternative perspective (Exercise 6.7) would be most helpful. She also realized, though, that her worry about what other people thought of her was a long-standing problem, and so she decided to work on that part of her anxiety problem by following the specialized cognitive therapy for worry program presented in Chapter 11.

Hannah realized that she needed to develop a more detailed plan for how she would carry out each of the interventions listed on her Anxiety Work Plan. How, for example, would she go about gathering evidence for and against her automatic anxious thought "I've offended my friend, and now she won't like me"? She decided she could write down from memory the times she had had conversations with people over the last month and whether these conversations had had a good or bad outcome (e.g., "Did the person refuse to speak to me afterward?"). Also, how many times had she been told she had offended another person? She could even do a one-

Planning your treatment involves knowing how you're going to work on each anxiety symptom. Use the cognitive and behavioral skills you learned in Chapters 6 and 7 as tools for taking a cognitive therapy approach to reducing your anxiety.

time survey of a few close friends and family and ask whether they thought she tended to offend people. Then, over the next 2 weeks, she would monitor the outcome of her casual conversations with people. Like Hannah, you will need an implementation plan for how you will carry out the interventions listed on your Anxiety Work Plan. Review the relevant sections in Chapters 6 and 7 to help with developing your intervention strategy.

Step 3: Create a Self-Help Schedule

In the third column of the Anxiety Work Plan, write down a schedule for doing the interventions listed for each target symptom. Try to be as specific as possible—note when you will do the intervention, how often, where, and for how long. Review Chapter 4 if you need to be reminded of the best way to do the self-help exercises. You could even enter reminders to do a particular intervention into your Day-Timer or smartphone. Hannah, for example, decided that coffee breaks and lunchtime were particularly good times to work on her anxiety at work. She decided that at least once a day she would initiate casual conversation lasting at least 5 minutes at these times. Be creative in thinking how you can fit times to work on your anxiety into your busy day. **Remember, the more work you do on anxiety, the quicker and better the results.** Procrastination and neglect are the enemies of anxiety reduction!

> Develop a weekly schedule for working on your anxiety. Be clear on what you are working on, when, where, and for how long. To overcome anxiety, you need to be committed to your plan.

Step 4: Record the Outcome

The final column of Worksheet 8.1 provides an opportunity for you to keep some notes on whether the interventions were helpful for each anxiety symptom. Did you experience a reduction in anxiety? Were the interventions difficult or easier to do than you expected? Did any experiences with the interventions seem to have a significant impact on your anxiety? Do you need more practice working on this anxiety symptom, or can you move on to the next target symptom?

Hannah, for example, found gathering evidence and decatastrophizing especially helpful in correcting her anxious thought "I've offended my friend, and now she won't like me." She was able to develop a normalization card that reminded her that it's impossible to know what people really think of you. How would you know if

> At the end of each week, evaluate the success of the intervention exercises you've done so you know what is and is not working for you and can make adjustments in your cognitive therapy program.

something you said was a little offensive or terribly offensive? And does it really matter in the end? If the person is still friendly toward you, any offense committed must be considered trivial, inconsequential to the person. Hannah considered this intervention highly significant in reducing her anxiety about offending people. The outcome column in the Anxiety Work Plan should be completed weekly, after you've had a chance to work on a particular anxiety symptom over several days.

Beth's Anxiety Work Plan

We introduced Beth in Chapter 5, where you had a chance to see how she filled out the Anxiety Profile. On page 159 you can see enough of Beth's Anxiety Work Plan to provide you with an illustration (space limitations prevent us from reproducing the entire worksheet).

Note that Beth's Anxiety Work Plan is based on her Anxiety Profile, just as yours should be. Also notice that some of the interventions Beth scheduled addressed more than one anxiety symptom. You'll often find that an exercise such as exposure or a behavioral experiment will target an anxiety trigger, some form of anxious thinking, and a coping response such as escape or avoidance. The fact that they can deal with several elements of your anxiety makes some intervention exercises more powerful than others.

Now that you've completed your Anxiety Work Plan, it's time to get started. Use the Worksheets in Chapters 6 and 7 to help you engage in your intervention tasks. Also look back at the work you completed in Chapters 1–5 to give you ideas for what situations, thoughts, and behaviors need to be changed to reduce your anxiety.

Specialized Cognitive Therapy

You have learned about the basic cognitive therapy approach to anxiety in the first eight chapters of this workbook. The program of change we've described will be effective for most types of anxiety. However, in the last 20 years we've learned a great deal about special forms of anxiety, especially panic attacks, social anxiety, and worry. Special versions of cognitive therapy have been developed that target unique features of these forms of anxiety. You will find these specialized types of cognitive therapy in the last three chapters of the workbook.

You may find that you end up wanting to use these specialized cognitive therapy approaches if you have a particularly intense or long-standing problem with panic attacks, social anxiety, or worry. Sometimes fear of panic, intense anxiety around others, or chronic worry remains a problem after people do the standard cognitive therapy exercises, particularly when they've been struggling with anxiety for years. Everything in the specialized chapters builds on what you've learned so far. You will

Beth's Anxiety Work Plan

Targeted Anxiety Symptom	Intervention Exercises	Self-Help Schedule	Outcome
PART I. ANXIETY TRIGGERS (situations, etc.)			
1. Going to the supermarket alone and running into a neighbor.	Develop exposure plan and normalization card (Exercises 7.1 and 7.2).	First go to distant supermarket at least twice and then go to neighborhood supermarket three times a week at peak hours; stay each time for at least 20 minutes. Work on this for 2 weeks.	Completed; can enter neighborhood grocery store with only mild anxiety; exposure highly effective.
2. Initiate phone call to an old friend I've not spoken to for months.	Develop exposure plan and normalization card (Exercises 7.1 and 7.2).	First send e-mail to old friend and ask for a good time to call; then make the call before end of week. Talk for at least 10 minutes.	In progress
3. Receive e-mail that I'm to speak at the end-of-the-week staff meeting.	Engage in worry interventions (Chapter 11).	For the next four evenings I will spend at least 30 minutes after supper working on my worry about the meeting. When worry enters my mind during the day, I will put it on the agenda for the evening worry session.	Planned

Targeted Anxiety Symptom	Intervention Exercises	Self-Help Schedule	Outcome
PART II. THREAT EVALUATION (anxious thinking)			
4. I am feeling hot and sweaty; people will notice I'm anxious. (physical evaluation)	Use thought monitoring, (Exercise 6.2), evidence gathering (Exercise 6.3), cost–benefit (Exercise 6.4), and develop alternative (Exercise 6.7).	Have at least two conversations a day with coworkers; speak to cashiers once a day; try to exhibit some anxiety. Do this one week; record anxious thoughts and then complete worksheets for 30 minutes in the evening.	Completed; no longer believe this; have thought only occasionally
5. People will see that I am perspiring and be disgusted by me. (automatic threat thought)	Use evidence gathering (Exercise 6.3), decatastrophizing (Exercise 6.5), normalization card (Exercise 6.8), and behavioral experiment (Worksheet 7.5).	Wear sweater to next staff meeting and sit next to heater. Record whether anyone notices that I am hot; make comment to someone that I feel hot. In evening, complete worksheets on anxious thoughts related to this assignment.	In progress
6. If I'm anxious around people, I am more likely to embarrass myself. (anxiety belief)	Use thought monitoring, (Exercise 6.2), evidence gathering (Exercise 6.3), cost–benefit (Exercise 6.4), developing alternative perspective (Exercise 6.7), and do behavioral experiment (Worksheet 7.5).	At least three times a week, have conversations with unfamiliar people, speak up at a meeting, make a phone call that generates anxiety. Record evidence that I embarrassed myself during these activities. Use worksheets to correct anxious thinking within 1 hour after completing an assignment.	Planned

Targeted Anxiety Symptom	Intervention Exercises	Self-Help Schedule	Outcome
7. Catastrophize about sweat, emotional reasoning, jump to conclusions (thinking errors)	Monitor thinking errors (Exercise 6.2), identify and correct (Exercise 6.6).	Each time I do an assignment, look for errors in my thinking.	In progress
PART III. COPING RESPONSES (avoidance, safety seeking, etc.)			
8. I am socially awkward and generally quite unfriendly. (helplessness beliefs)	Develop a normalization card (Exercises 6.8 and 7.1) and then practice exposure to social interaction (Exercise 7.2).	Initiate at least three conversations this week, one with an unfamiliar person; evaluate my social performance; gather evidence for and against a poor performance.	Completed; very successful. Was surprised at my conversational skills despite feeling some anxiety.
9. Avoid all social gatherings if at all possible. (avoidance)	Engage in repeated exposure to a hierarchy of social interaction (Exercise 7.2)	Each day I must engage in at least one task from my exposure hierarchy (Worksheet 7.3).	In progress; have already conquered tasks in the moderate anxiety range.
10. Carry Ativan at all times and will take a pill if I anticipate a social event. (safety seeking)	Gradually hold off taking an Ativan for social interactions and keep the Ativan in less and less accessible places (Worksheet 7.6).	The next week, leave the Ativan in my desk drawer at work rather than carrying it around with me.	In progress; keep Ativan in car, desk drawer, or medicine cabinet at home. Still a way to go before I can stop the medication.
11. What if I end up alone and friendless because no one wants to be around a self-conscious, uptight woman? (anxious worry)	Do the worry exercises described in chapter.	I will schedule three times a week a 30-minute worry exposure session and engage in cognitive skills that target worry (see Ch. 11). I will hold off doing this until I've made progress on other anxiety symptoms.	Planned

find that some of the interventions have been modified to deal with specific aspects of panic attacks, social anxiety, and worry. So the work you completed so far will be invaluable as you proceed to the specialized chapters.

Maintaining Your Gains

Fear and anxiety have a nasty habit of returning! Even if you've made great progress using this workbook, and you've achieved many of the goals listed in Worksheet 1.1, anxiety can come back to bite you. As we've pointed out repeatedly, fear and anxiety are a normal part of life. But once anxiety has crossed the line from normal to excessive, it can do so again. So you need to prepare for the possibility of falling back into old ways of thinking, behaving, and feeling.

The best way to maintain your gains is to know the signs that your anxiety is getting out of hand:

- **Avoidance creeps back.** You start avoiding some of the anxiety triggers from the past.

- **You become less tolerant of feeling anxious.** You're more bothered by feeling anxious and begin taking steps to avoid anxious feelings and symptoms.

- **Worry increases.** You are thinking more about anxiety and find yourself increasingly worried about the possibility of becoming anxious.

- **Your belief in threat and catastrophe returns.** You find yourself more accepting of the automatic thoughts of danger, catastrophe, and the worst-case scenario.

- **Safety seeking increases.** You resume taking antianxiety medication or engage in other activities to exert greater control over anxiety.

- **Anxiety interferes in your life more.** You notice that you're isolating yourself more or you're having trouble sleeping or concentrating at work. You may feel more depressed or irritable. Anxiety is creeping back into your life and eating away at your quality of living.

There are two approaches you can take to a return of fear. First, you can review the workbook. Go back to your worksheets, redo some of the exercises, and reapply the interventions. You'll probably find that the same approaches that were successful in the past will be helpful again. In fact we find that the interventions work more quickly the second or third time around. You probably will need to work on your anxiety much less intensely this second time.

You also might benefit from working with a cognitive behavior therapist. Many people find they can go only so far on their own and need the guidance and expertise of a therapist. The workbook itself may prove much more effective if you were in therapy. There's no magic formula for determining who needs therapy for anxiety, so let's keep it simple: Go back to the workbook if you were satisfied with the progress you made with the workbook alone the first time around. Consult a therapist if you weren't completely satisfied. The Resources at the back of the book can steer you to websites and organizations that will help you find qualified cognitive therapy.

Know the signs that anxiety is returning, and when you spot them, don't delay in revisiting your Anxiety Work Plan and redoing some of the critical cognitive and behavioral interventions that you found so effective. Also consider whether working with a qualified therapist might give your cognitive therapy program a needed boost.

CHAPTER SUMMARY

■ Having a cognitive therapy work plan will keep you focused on what needs to be changed to overcome anxiety and lessen that "swamped feeling" often experienced with emotional change.

■ Taking the time to construct a personal Anxiety Work Plan will maximize the effectiveness of the intervention skills discussed in this workbook.

■ Use Worksheet 8.1 to develop a unique Anxiety Work Plan that focuses on your experience of anxiety. The work plan is organized like the Anxiety Profile (Worksheet 5.9) so they can be used together to plan out your cognitive therapy program.

■ At any time in your intervention, you should be working on one situational trigger, an anxious thought, and a coping response. Use Worksheet 8.1 to describe the anxiety symptom, the intervention exercises you'll apply to that symptom, an implementation schedule, and the outcome of your efforts.

■ The specialized cognitive therapies in Chapters 9–11 are particularly helpful for those with intense and long-standing problems with panic attacks, social anxiety, and/or worry.

■ Expect fear and anxiety to return. The cognitive and behavioral interventions described in this workbook can be reapplied effectively to the return of anxiety. Also consider whether you might benefit from the guidance and expertise of a cognitive behavior therapist.

9

Defeating Panic and Avoidance

This chapter is especially relevant for you if:

- You've been working on your anxiety using the Anxiety Work Plan you created in Chapter 8 but you're still having significant problems with panic attacks.

- You reduced your anxiety significantly using Chapters 1–8 but you are still avoiding or trying to control anxiety because you are still afraid of having panic attacks.

- Despite some progress you are still very attentive to the physical symptoms of anxiety and are afraid to let yourself get too anxious.

- After working through Chapters 1–8 you're experiencing a return of anxiety in the form of panic attacks or fear of panic.

Lucia, age 35, had her first panic attack 6 months after her father recovered from a serious heart attack. The heart attack took the whole family by surprise—Dad had no cardiac risk factors, was in excellent health, and exercised religiously. Very close to her parents, Lucia took time off from work and from taking care of her three children to help her father get back on his feet and back to his own job. She was at work on the day she later described as "the worst day of my life." It had been a particularly stressful day filled with deadlines that needed to be met and numerous interruptions that kept putting her behind.

Suddenly, out of the blue, Lucia felt a crushing pain in her chest, her heart started beating rapidly, she felt hot and flushed, and she couldn't seem to get enough air. She loosened the top of her blouse and noticed that her hand was trembling. Lucia tried to get up from her seat but felt a weakness throughout her body. Her knees began to buckle, and she had to hold on to her desk to keep from falling. She felt dizzy and somewhat disoriented. All she could think about was her father's heart attack.

Was she now experiencing the same thing? "Is this what it feels like to have a heart attack?" Although it was only a few minutes before the symptoms began to subside, time seemed to drag.

Lucia eventually made it to the washroom, where she bathed her face in cold water. Still, there was a lingering heaviness in her chest, and she seemed to struggle to get enough air. She returned to her desk, but she was much too worried and keyed up to work. She told her supervisor she was not well and left the office early. Instead of driving straight home, Lucia stopped at the emergency room of her local hospital, where a battery of tests turned up nothing that could account for her symptoms. The ER physician concluded that Lucia had experienced a panic attack. He gave her a couple of Ativan and told her to see her family physician.

That was 3 years ago. Since then Lucia's world has turned upside down. She now experiences almost constant anxiety. She worries about having another panic attack. The once energetic, competent wife, mother, and employee has cut back so much on her activities that she now practically confines herself to work and home. She refuses to travel outside her city, avoids public places, can't cross bridges, and is afraid to be left alone at night. She is preoccupied with her physical state and is now afraid that she's going crazy. She has tried various medications, but the only thing that seems to work is a tranquilizer, and even that calms her down for only a couple of hours. It's been ages since she got a good night's sleep.

Lucia's husband is losing patience with her refusal to leave the house except for work, and their arguments have only added to her depression and discouragement that she can't seem to beat the anxiety. A few weeks ago, after a particularly intense argument, she wondered whether her family would be better off if she ended her life. Relating this incident to her family physician at the next appointment, Lucia was referred to a therapist for treatment of panic disorder and agoraphobia.

Lucia was ready to try anything. For 3 years she'd felt as if the fear of panic attacks was holding her hostage. She was ready to be liberated. You may feel the same way, especially if you've tried the general cognitive therapy program laid out in the preceding chapters but still avoid participating fully in your life for fear of having another panic attack. In this chapter we'll show you how to customize the interventions you learned in earlier chapters to address panic in particular. Just as you created an Anxiety Profile in Chapter 5, you'll create a panic profile here. Then we'll show you how to use (1) a specific adaptation of the decatastrophizing you learned in Chapter 6 that can significantly reduce the frequency and fear of panic attacks and (2) exposure to reduce avoidance of panic triggers.

Panic Attacks: The "Tsunami" of Anxiety

If you're to benefit from the interventions aimed specifically at reducing panic, it's important to make sure panic is what you're dealing with. If you've experienced a panic attack, you'll probably never forget it. Maybe you were feeling only a little on edge or even quite calm, when suddenly you were caught off guard by a wave of intense anxiety. Having what we call a "spontaneous panic attack" feels like a "tsunami of anxiety" has swept over you.

A *panic attack* is defined as:

a distinct period or episode of intense fear or discomfort that builds suddenly, peaks briefly, and is characterized by a number of physical sensations and frightening cognitions. Typically panic attacks last between 5 and 20 minutes.

According to DSM-IV-TR[14] of the American Psychiatric Association, a "full-blown" panic attack is a discrete period of intense fear or discomfort that peaks quickly (i.e., within 10 minutes at most) and includes four or more of the following symptoms:

- Palpitations, pounding heart, or accelerated heart rate
- Sweating
- Trembling or shaking
- Sensations of shortness of breath or smothering
- Feeling of choking
- Chest pain or discomfort
- Nausea or abdominal distress
- Feeling dizzy, unsteady, lightheaded, or faint
- Derealization (feelings of unreality) or depersonalization (being detached from oneself)
- Fear of losing control or going crazy
- Paresthesias (numbness or tingling sensations)
- Chills or hot flushes*

Do these symptoms sound familiar to you? If you've had at least two unexpected panic attacks characterized by such symptoms, you may qualify for a diagnosis of panic disorder. But panic attacks also occur in a variety of other anxiety disorders, so a specific diagnosis of panic disorder isn't necessary for you to be plagued by, and be motivated to address, panic attacks.

---

*Reprinted with permission from the *Diagnostic and Statistical Manual of Mental Disorders, Fourth Edition, Text Revision* (p. 432). Copyright 2000 by the American Psychiatric Association.

Four Significant Features of Panic

There are four characteristics of panic that you should know about, because they each play an important role in the interventions designed to reduce panic attacks and panic disorder.

Certain Situations Trigger Panic

Interestingly, although at least two panic attacks must come "out of the blue" to be part of panic disorder, most people who have panic attacks know full well that panic is usually triggered by particular situations, such as being in public places, social situations, being alone, having to perform in front of an audience, and the like. **In fact, a person with panic attacks learns quickly what situations are likely to trigger a panic attack and thus avoids these situations.** Lucia soon learned that unfamiliar situations heightened her anxiety and the risk of a panic attack, so she restricted herself more and more to home and work.

> What are the situations that you fear will trigger a panic attack? How often do you avoid these situations for fear of panic? In the blanks below, list the situations that you fear will most likely trigger a panic attack. Next to each, note whether you always avoid this situation or avoid it only sometimes.
>
> 1. _____
>
> 2. _____
>
> 3. _____
>
> 4. _____
>
> 5. _____

Panic Causes Preoccupation with the Physical Symptoms

People who suffer panic not only learn to avoid situations they fear will trigger an attack but also become so frightened of the physical sensations of panic that they focus constantly on their physical state, monitoring their body for unexplained physical feelings throughout the day. Because of her fear of a heart attack, Lucia became preoccupied with pains, tightness, and pressure in her chest. She even started to take her pulse periodically to ensure she wasn't having heart palpitations. It was as if she had lost all confidence in her cardiovascular system, fearful it would go awry and her heart would start beating erratically.

> What physical symptoms scare you most? Are there certain bodily sensations that you tend to monitor for fear they signal an impending panic attack? Write down the two or three bodily sensations that you are most conscious of because they signal the possibility of a panic attack:
>
> 1. _____
>
> 2. _____
>
> 3. _____

Catastrophizing Is at the Core of Panic

For individuals who suffer from repeated panic attacks, panic represents a catastrophe! The types of catastrophic thinking most common in panic disorder are:

- Fear of dying from a heart attack, suffocation, brain tumor, or the like
- Fear of losing control, "going crazy," or causing extreme embarrassment
- Fear of having more frequent, intense, and uncontrolled panic attacks

It's not that you necessarily believe you're having a heart attack or are going insane. The catastrophic thinking occurs automatically, as a question, like "What if this feeling of not getting enough air gets worse and I can't breathe?" Also, the catastrophic thinking is normally linked to particular bodily sensations such as chest tightness and heart attacks, nausea and uncontrollable vomiting, dizziness or light-headedness, and losing control or going crazy. At the center of cognitive therapy for panic is the assertion that *the catastrophic misinterpretation of bodily sensations* is the core problem in panic attacks.[4,5,32] Lucia connected chest tightness and heart palpitations with her panic attacks. Whenever she felt some unexplained pressure in her chest, she automatically thought "What's wrong with my chest? It doesn't feel right to me. Am I getting anxious or stressed out? Is this putting too much pressure on my

> Whenever you experience unwanted bodily sensations related to panic, what is the worst possible outcome (catastrophe) you fear? Write down the most frequent catastrophic misinterpretation (the worst possible outcome) that lingers in the back of your mind when you feel panicky.
>
> _____
>
> _____

heart? How would I know if I'm having a heart attack? What if this leads to a full-blown panic attack right here in front of all these people?"

Strategies Intended to Prevent Panic Start to Take Over Daily Life

Finally, panic attacks are so dreaded that people usually develop particular strategies aimed at preventing further attacks. They strive to feel safe and comfortable because they believe this is the best defense against panic. Consequently escape, avoidance, and safety-seeking or anxiety control behaviors come to dominate their life. Not only did Lucia avoid places that made her feel more anxious, but she always had her Ativan close by in case she needed it, and she would go to certain places only if her husband went with her. Chapter 3 listed typical cognitive and behavioral safety-seeking measures, and in Chapter 5 you recorded your own coping responses in Part III of your Anxiety Profile (Worksheet 5.9), based on having examined them in detail in Worksheets 5.6 and 5.7. If you need to remind yourself of how you usually try to avoid triggers of panic, go back to those earlier chapters before filling in the following box.

When you're afraid you might have a panic attack, what do you do to avoid or minimize the possibility of an escalation in anxiety that could result in panic?

1. _____

2. _____

3. _____

4. _____

Are You Ready to Tackle Panic?

Between 13% and 33% of the general population report having experienced at least one panic attack in the last year,[33,34] but whether you decide to address panic separately via this chapter will probably depend on how severely it's interfering in your life. Worksheet 9.1 presents a checklist of statements you should review to determine whether your experience with panic attacks may be a clinical problem. This is not a checklist for diagnosing panic disorder, but it may help you gauge the severity of your panic and decide whether it's time to take further action.

Panic attacks come in different forms as well as varying levels of severity. Many people with panic disorder will wake up in the middle of the night with a panic attack (called *nocturnal panic attacks*), and most people with panic experience frequent limited-symptom panic (mini-attacks) that involves only one or two physical

Panic Self-Diagnostic Checklist

Instructions: Read each statement below and decide whether it applies to you. If you answered "yes" to a majority of these statements, it's likely that panic attacks are a serious clinical problem for you.

Question	Yes	No
1. I have full-blown panic attacks several times a week.		
2. My panic attacks typically involve several physical symptoms listed on page 166.		
3. I have become frightened of having panic attacks.		
4. I tend to avoid a number of common, everyday situations for fear of panic.		
5. Whenever I feel a little anxious, I worry it will escalate into a panic attack.		
6. I find myself preoccupied with monitoring my body for unexpected physical sensations and symptoms.		
7. I am increasingly relying on other people to accompany me so I'll feel less anxious.		
8. Whenever I have an unexplained body sensation or physical symptom, my initial reaction is to assume the worst possible outcome.		
9. I find it very difficult to think more rationally when I feel panicky.		
10. I try hard to keep myself calm so I don't become too stressed out and anxious.		
11. I have become much less tolerant with feeling anxious.		
12. I seem less capable of correcting my initial catastrophic misinterpretation of unexplained physical sensations.		
13. I feel like I've become too emotional and concerned about losing control.		
14. Fear of panic is significantly interfering in my work, school, leisure, and quality of life.		
15. My family and friends are losing patience with my struggle with panic and my avoidance of everyday situations.		

Is panic holding you back, reducing your quality of life and fulfillment of important life goals? Are you ready for a different approach to your panic? Cognitive therapy is all about giving you the tools to handle panic more effectively so that panic stops "handling" you!

symptoms but significant apprehension and avoidance. The cognitive therapy approach presented in this chapter can be helpful for all these forms of panic. Its goal is **to normalize the panic experience—reduce its frequency, severity, and duration so that panic attacks play no greater role in your life than they do for the millions of people who have only occasional "nonclinical" panic attacks.**

Fear of Fear

The energetic, adventurous, "full of life" person that Lucia's friends knew has become timid, cautious, and worried since she had her first panic attack. Anxiety has a stranglehold on Lucia's life. Although Lucia's emotional conundrum was complicated, in many respects it all boiled down to a fear of being anxious, or "fear of fear." She became increasingly worried and intolerant of any physical symptoms of anxiety, especially any sensations involving her chest or heart. She became preoccupied with not being anxious and with maintaining a state of calm and safety. Her ultimate fear was that anxiety might escalate into panic or, even worse, overtax her heart and cause a heart attack.

In Chapter 3 we introduced the concept of *anxiety sensitivity* as an important feature of the anxious mind. Heightened anxiety sensitivity is defined as:

> *fear of experiencing the physical symptoms of anxiety (heart palpitations, nausea, chest pains, breathlessness, etc.) because one believes these symptoms will lead to severe negative consequences (a full-blown panic attack, loss of control, extreme embarrassment, serious medical illness, etc.).*[35–37]

Heightened anxiety sensitivity plays a particularly important role in persistent panic states and could be a major reason that you're still suffering panic after having used the interventions earlier in this book. A person with high anxiety sensitivity who experiences, let's say, a slight feeling "of not being able to get enough air" immediately reacts by imposing the most negative construction on the feeling: "What if this feeling gets worse and I start to suffocate?" The person with low anxiety sensitivity experiences the same breathless sensation but immediately is more accepting of the feeling because she assumes a benign consequence: "I've had this feeling before, and it's nothing. Just take a couple of deep breaths and get back to work." There is evidence that anxiety sensitivity is an enduring personality characteristic that increases one's risk or vulnerability for developing a panic disorder.[37] High anxiety sensitivity fuels panic attacks by:

- Increasing the likelihood that a person automatically makes a catastrophic misinterpretation of an unexplained bodily sensation

- Decreasing a person's acceptance of her anxiety and reinforcing her determination to control anxious feelings

- Encouraging the avoidance of anxiety-related triggers and safety-seeking behaviors

Do you suffer from high anxiety sensitivity? Knowing whether you are prone to anxiety sensitivity is important to effective cognitive therapy for panic. Worksheet 9.2 lists a few core beliefs you can use to determine whether you have high anxiety sensitivity.

> In cognitive therapy, evaluation and correction of anxiety sensitivity beliefs play an important role in reducing the frequency and severity of panic attacks.

The Panic-Stricken Mind

Lucia knew she was not having a heart attack when she felt pressure or tightness in her chest. She realized it was probably just anxiety or stress. But she couldn't seem to stop herself from thinking the *what ifs*: "What if this time the chest tightness is due to problems with my heart?" "What if the symptoms persist and develop into a full-blown panic attack?" "What if I lose complete control and the symptoms don't go away?" Even though Lucia had now experienced the physical symptoms of anxiety dozens of times and the worst thing that had happened was heightened anxiety, she couldn't help thinking about these worst-case scenarios. These *what ifs* were the first thoughts that popped into her mind when she noticed the unwanted physical sensations. They were her first apprehensive thoughts, and they always focused on some mental, emotional, or medical catastrophe. Lucia had developed a *panic mind-set,* and it was this way of thinking that was responsible for her continued problem with panic attacks.

The way you think about the physical symptoms of anxiety is pivotal to the development and persistence of panic attacks. Cognitive therapy focuses on modifying the panic-stricken mind to eliminate fear of anxious feelings (i.e., anxiety sensitivity) and thereby reduce the frequency and intensity of panic episodes. The diagram on page 174 illustrates the cognitive model of panic attacks. There are four key elements in the "anatomy of a panic attack" that we target in therapy.

Hypervigilance

As we've explained, and as shown in the diagram, when you have frequent panic attacks you can become preoccupied with your physical state, frequently monitor-

Anxiety Sensitivity Beliefs

Instructions: Circle how much each of the following statements applies to you. If you circle "much" or "very much" to three or more items, it may be that anxiety sensitivity is an important factor in your panic attacks.

Statements	Very Little	A Little	Some	Much	Very Much
1. I am afraid of my heart beating quickly because I tend to think something could be terribly wrong.	0	1	2	3	4
2. When my stomach feels queasy or upset, I start to worry that I might become sick.	0	1	2	3	4
3. When I feel unexpected chest tightness or pains, my initial fearful thought is whether this could be a sign or symptom of a heart attack.	0	1	2	3	4
4. When I feel like I am not breathing properly, I tend to think this is serious and could lead to suffocation.	0	1	2	3	4
5. When my throat feels tight, I seriously wonder if I could choke to death.	0	1	2	3	4
6. It is important to keep myself calm and relaxed as much as possible.	0	1	2	3	4
7. I try to control my anxiety so I don't look nervous to other people.	0	1	2	3	4
8. I don't like feeling physically aroused or excited.	0	1	2	3	4
9. I am concerned that physical arousal or stress could get out of hand and cause a panic attack.	0	1	2	3	4
10. I am quite preoccupied with how I am feeling physically and whether I am starting to feel anxious.	0	1	2	3	4

Note. These statements are intended to indicate whether a person has a tendency toward high anxiety sensitivity. An accurate assessment of anxiety sensitivity can be done only by a qualified mental health professional using a standardized anxiety sensitivity measure.[38]

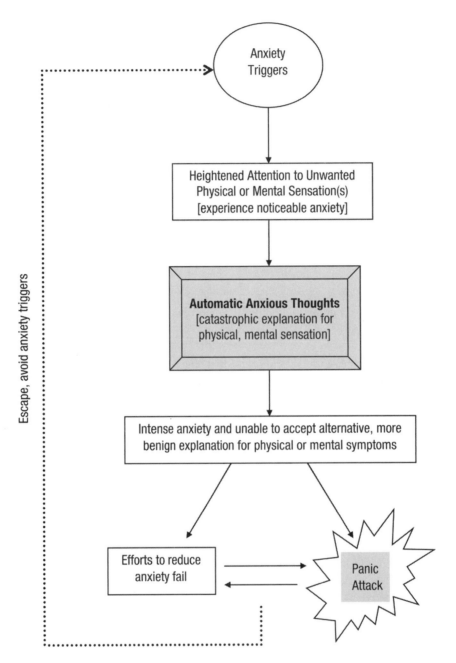

The cognitive model of panic.

ing your bodily functions for unwanted or unexplained physical sensations. That is, you develop a state of "physical hypervigilance." As long as a physical symptom, like chest tightness, difficulty breathing, dizziness, or nausea, can be explained or is expected (e.g., "I just walked up a flight of stairs, so of course I am out of breath"), you feel somewhat better, although the remote possibility of the worst-case scenario may still linger in the back of your mind. If the physical sensation is unexpected and inexplicable (e.g., "I'm just sitting at my desk; I shouldn't be feeling like I can't get enough air"), apprehension sets in immediately because catastrophic thinking takes over. You think: "This is not normal," "Why am I feeling this way?" or "Something's not right with me." Lucia, for example, became hypersensitive about the functioning of her heart and lungs. She became preoccupied with any sensation in her chest, her heart rate, whether she was breathing properly. She even got to the point of frequently taking her pulse throughout the day to see whether her heart rate was elevated. Whenever she was aware of an unwanted physical sensation, she immediately became apprehensive, asking, "What's wrong with me?"

> People who suffer frequent panic attacks often develop a hypersensitivity to the first physical signs of anxiety, which causes them to feel perpetually anxious about their physical state. Cognitive therapy for panic focuses on "turning down" this excessive body self-monitoring.

Catastrophizing

Earlier we said that *catastrophic misinterpretation of unexplained physical sensations* is at the core of panic attacks, which is why this element is highlighted right in the center of the diagram: it's the pivotal event in creating panic. Hypervigilance can produce an immediate, automatic thought of the worst-case scenario: "What if I'm having a heart attack? What if I lose control and this develops into a panic attack? What if I'm going crazy?" In panic, the catastrophic thinking involves exaggerating the likelihood and severity of this worst possible outcome, such as overestimating the probability that heart palpitations reflect an underlying heart problem. When asked about chest tightness, Lucia completely overestimated the number of times it's linked to cardiac dysfunction.

> Cognitive therapy can teach you how to counter this "catastrophic misinterpretation of physical sensations" so that anxious feelings do not escalate into panic.

Certain physical sensations tend to lead to particular misinterpretations. A list of typical misinterpretations of bodily sensations is presented in Table 9.1. Do you experience any of these ways of thinking about your physical sensations when you're feeling anxious?

Failure to Correct

We've all experienced unexpected, spontaneous physical sensations and possibly even occasionally entertained a catastrophic interpretation ("Could this be something serious?"). But where most people tend to correct that initial anxious thought—to reevaluate the bodily sensation as a random, benign, and inconsequential occurrence—the ability to do so comes very hard to you if you suffer frequent panic attacks. It's as if your first automatic anxious thought ("Something could be terribly wrong with me")

TABLE 9.1. **Examples of Catastrophic Thinking and Associated Bodily Sensations**

Internal sensation	Automatic anxious (catastrophic) thoughts
Chest tightness, pain, heart palpitations	• "Something's wrong with my heart." • "Could I be having a heart attack?" • "Am I putting too much stress on my heart?"
Breathlessness, smothering sensation, irregular breathing	• "I'm not getting enough air." • "What if I start to suffocate?" • "I can't breathe deeply enough."
Dizziness, lightheadedness, faintness	• "I'm losing control." • "Am I going crazy?" • "Could this be a symptom of a brain tumor?"
Nausea, abdominal cramps	• "What if I become really sick and start vomiting?"
Numbness, tingling in extremities	• "Am I having a stroke?" • "Am I losing control and going crazy?"
Restlessness, tension, agitation	• "Is this the beginning of a full-blown panic attack?" • "Am I losing complete control of my emotions?" • "I'm overly stressed."
Feeling shaky, trembling	[same interpretation as previous symptoms]
Forgetfulness, inattention, loss of concentration	• "I'm losing control over my mental functioning." • "Something is terribly wrong with me." • "What if I have a serious loss of intellectual ability?"
Feelings of unreality, depersonalization	• "Could this develop into a seizure?" • "Is this a sign that I am going insane, that I am having a nervous breakdown?"

Note. Based on *Understanding and Treating Panic Disorder: Cognitive-Behavioural Approaches* by Steven Taylor. Chichester, UK: Wiley.

takes off on its own, like a runaway freight train, unchecked by more rational think-ing. Lucia, for example, couldn't seem to escape doubts about her heart whenever she felt unexplained sensations in her chest. She tried to tell herself "Oh, it's nothing; it's probably just indigestion," or "It's just a random physical sensation," but she couldn't seem to accept these alternatives. She was drawn back to the *what if*s: "What if some-thing really is wrong with my heart?" Lucia tried to counter catastrophized thinking with more rational explanations, but they were weak and ineffectual against her "all-powerful catastrophizing," which seemed to paralyze her.

We all experience daily fluctuations in breathing, heart rate, gastrointestinal and neurological sensations, muscle aches and pains that result from the changing demands on our body. It would be unrealistic to expect our bodies to function perfectly, given all of these demands on it. Are you inclined to be too hasty, jumping to conclusions (a cognitive error) about what might be causing a particular physical sensation? Listed below are some alternative, more benign causes of physical sensations that are common and expected in healthy people. Compare these causes to the catastrophic scenarios in Table 9.1 and ask yourself which you find more believable for the bodily sensations you repeatedly experience.

- Increased physical activity, exercise
- Fatigue, lack of energy
- Consumption of or withdrawal from a stimulant like caffeine
- Consumption of or withdrawal from alcohol or prescription medication
- Consequence of heightened stress or general anxiety
- Disturbance in balance
- Changes in the immediate environment such as lighting, temperature, etc.
- Heightened preoccupation or monitoring of one's physical state
- Observing or hearing about physical symptoms in others
- Indigestion or other digestive reactions to food intake
- Bowel irregularity, motility, or gut contractions
- Allergic reactions
- Increased frustration, irritability, anger
- Premenstrual symptoms
- Strenuous dieting, hunger
- Spontaneous fluctuations in physical function

Cognitive therapy can strengthen your reappraisal capabilities so you can correct your tendency to catastrophize and learn to interrupt the vicious cycle of panic.

Safety Seeking and Control

A natural consequence of "thinking the worst" is feeling that you're losing control. As the physical symptoms intensify and you become more and more anxious, it seems as if you're losing complete control of mind and body. You become convinced that the situation is intolerable—something must be done. So naturally, automatically you seek to gain control, to escape the situation, to calm yourself and seek a place of safety. As discussed in Chapter 3, escape, avoidance, and the search for safety become the *modus operandi* of the anxious mind. In panic disorder this will include any strategy that helps you relax to reduce a feared physical sensation—consume alcohol, take medication, meditate, and so on. Situations thought to trigger anxiety are avoided, and often you learn to flee at the first signs of anxiety. This is why agoraphobia is often a complication of panic disorder. Lucia came to realize that public places like grocery stores, malls, and movie theaters heightened her anxiety level and increased the risk of panic attacks, so she started avoiding these places. In a few months she found herself practically housebound.

The search for safety, escape, and avoidance are major contributors to the persistence of anxiety and panic, which is why the elimination of avoidance and safety-seeking responses is such an important component of cognitive therapy for panic. In preparation for the sections to follow, look back at how you filled in Part III of your Anxiety Profile (Worksheet 5.9). Then transfer the situations you avoid for fear of panic attacks and the various strategies you employ in an effort to control or minimize feared physical sensations to Worksheet 9.3.

> Cognitive therapy teaches you how to relinquish futile efforts at control and safety seeking by adopting a more positive approach to the physical manifestations of anxiety and panic.

Your Panic Profile

Know your panic! One of the worst features of panic attacks is their spontaneous, unexpected, and totally inexplicable nature. Panickers often spend a great deal of time worrying about panic attacks, trying to figure out what is safe and what is dangerous and how they can avoid risk of another panic attack. Unfortunately, much of this attempt to "control panic" is futile at best and positively destructive at worst. Instead one of the best defenses against panic is knowledge and understanding. This is why **getting to know your panic, educating yourself about your panic reaction,** is the very first step in cognitive treatment of panic attacks. We want to take the surprise out of panic. We want you to become so familiar with your panic-related thinking and behavior that it no longer feels foreign or intimidating to you. In the first few cognitive therapy sessions, Lucia learned about her own unique "vicious cycle of panic." She was surprised at how focused she had become on her physical functioning, how quickly she jumped to worst-case interpretations, and how many subtle safety-seeking responses she used in a typical day (e.g., always had her cell phone, bottled water, medication handy in case she felt unwell).

What is your vicious cycle of panic? The cognitive model of panic on page 174 shows the components of this vicious cycle. To know your panic, you need to plot out your panic cycle. One way to do this is to think back to some recent panic episodes or even your worst panic attack. But another very important tool in developing your panic profile is a panic log.

We've found that individuals with panic disorder can achieve significant reduc-

Avoided Situations and Control Strategies Associated with Panic Attacks

Avoided Situations (Triggers)	Physical Symptom Control Strategies
1.	1.
2.	2.
3.	3.
4.	4.
5.	5.
6.	6.
7.	7.
8.	8.
9.	9.
10.	10.
11.	11.
12.	12.

tions in the frequency of their panic attacks simply by keeping a panic log, for these reasons:

- You learn to slow down and catch the automatic catastrophic misinterpretations of physical symptoms that cause panic attacks.
- Your anxiety becomes less surprising and unexpected as you learn more about it.
- You will feel a greater sense of personal control over your anxiety the more you understand the anxiety process.
- It provides opportunities for you to document evidence that is contrary to your automatic catastrophic misinterpretations.

Self-Help Exercise 9.1. Using the Panic Log

Make multiple copies of the Weekly Panic and Acute Anxiety Log (Worksheet 9.4) and record all significant anxiety and panic episodes. Complete the panic log as accurately as possible and as soon after an anxiety episode as feasible. Do this until you have recorded a few panic or anxiety episodes that will provide enough information to fill out your panic profile, but know that the more information you gather on your panic attacks and record in your panic log, the more effective the panic log will become in reducing the frequency of panic attacks. So it's best to keep a panic log throughout the duration of your work on panic attacks.

Self-Help Exercise 9.2. Completing Your Panic Profile

Using Worksheet 9.5, write down all the situations that make you anxious, the unwanted physical sensations that make you uncomfortable, the worst outcome you dread, the more realistic explanation you can't seem to believe, your safety-seeking responses, and everything you tend to avoid to minimize the risk of panic. Besides the information you've gathered from your panic log, you can enter information from previous panic attacks. Use your Anxiety Profile (Worksheet 5.9) as a reminder.

Weekly Panic and Acute Anxiety Log

Dates: from: _____ to: _____

Instructions: Use this form to record any panic attacks, limited panic attacks, or acute anxiety episodes that you experienced in the past week. Try to complete the form as close to the anxiety episode as possible to increase the accuracy of your remarks.

Date, Time, and Duration of Episode	Situational Triggers (label E or UE*)	Severity of Anxiety (0–100; label FPA or AA*)	Main Physical or Mental Sensation That Bothered You	Automatic Catastrophic Interpretation of the Sensation	Possible Alternative, Benign Interpretation	Control Efforts and Safety Seeking
1.						
2.						
3.						
4.						
5.						

*E = expected to have panic in this situation; UE = panic occurred unexpectedly, completely out of the blue; FPA = full-blown panic attack; AA = acute anxiety episode.

Panic Profile

Instructions: Complete each of the sections below by referring to your panic log (Worksheet 9.4).

I. MAIN ANXIETY TRIGGERS RELATED TO PANIC
(i.e., situations, thoughts, sensations, expectations)

1. _____

2. _____

3. _____

4. _____

II. INITIAL PHYSICAL SENSATIONS

Physical sensations: _____

_____

Initial physical, mental sensations: _____

_____

Main physical, mental sensation (i.e., captures your attention): _____

_____

III. INTERPRETATION OF PHYSICAL SENSATIONS

Automatic, catastrophic interpretation: _____

_____

Alternative benign interpretation: _____

_____

IV: SAFETY-SEEKING AND CONTROL RESPONSES

Safety-seeking responses: _____

_____

Other attempts to control anxiety, prevent panic attacks: _____

_____

⅔ Troubleshooting Tips ⅗

Sometimes people have difficulty capturing their catastrophic interpretation of physical sensations when they start using panic logs. If this is the case for you, it might be helpful to review work you did earlier in this book: Look back at how you filled out Worksheets 2.2, 3.1, 3.4, 5.3, and 5.4. Others are reluctant to complete panic logs because they think it will draw attention to their panic and make it worse. In our experience the opposite happens—completing panic logs helps people understand their panic process and thus reduces panic symptoms. Remember that "knowledge is power" when it comes to beating panic, so don't give up on completing your panic log.

Once you've become familiar with monitoring your anxiety and panic episodes in the panic log and completed your panic profile, you're ready to use some of the cognitive and behavioral strategies discussed in Chapters 6 and 7. We have modified these interventions to more effectively target critical aspects of panic attacks.

> Creating a panic profile (knowing your panic) and learning to consistently monitor acute anxiety and panic using the panic log are critical: You must be able to use these two aspects of treatment before moving on to the more specialized intervention strategies developed to reduce the frequency and severity of panic.

Panic Reappraisal

Looking back on your panic log, you might be thinking "Why do I so easily jump to the catastrophic interpretation of these physical symptoms?" This was Lucia's response after spending a couple of weeks monitoring her anxiety and panic attacks. After she calmed down, she could easily see that her chest tightness was just a sign of stress or a random physical event. But in the panicky moment, she could not shake that initial catastrophic thought "What if I'm having a heart attack?" One of the main reasons the automatic anxious thought returns so easily is that we all tend to engage in emotional reasoning when anxious. It goes something like this: "I'm feeling anxious; therefore something awful must be about to happen." So Lucia would feel pressure or tightness in her chest, become anxious, and in the very process of being anxious the thought that something bad was about to happen to her became much more real. One of the best ways to correct this tendency to jump to catastrophic conclusions when anxious is to develop a more realistic, alternative explanation for unwanted bodily sensations and reactions.

Self-Help Exercise 9.3.
Creating Alternative Anti-Panic Explanations

For the next couple of weeks, use Worksheet 9.6 (or one of the forms from Chapter 6, Worksheet 6.3 or 6.5) to generate alternative explanations for your anxiety-related unwanted and uncomfortable physical, mental, or emotional sensations. Review the list of alternative interpretations on page 177 and select two or three possibilities if you need help in coming up with alternatives. Also on a blank sheet of paper, write down specific experiences—that is, evidence—that tend to support the alternative explanations. Attach your evidence sheet to Worksheet 9.6 so you can be reminded of the experiences you've had that support the alternative explanations for physical sensations.

Self-Help Exercise 9.4. Create an Anti-Panic Flashcard

Choose a time when you're not anxious and review your panic log (Worksheet 9.4) and your symptom reappraisal form (Worksheet 9.6). Select the main physical, mental, or emotional symptom that is most closely related to your panic attacks. Now review the list of benign interpretations from Worksheet 9.6 that offer the most likely explanation for the panic-related sensation. Elaborate on why you think this alternative interpretation is a better explanation. Now write the alternative interpretation on a 3" × 5" index card or load it into your mobile device. This will become your **Anti-Panic Flashcard.** You will need to read this flashcard repeatedly and each time write down why this explanation is true before your belief will start to shift from the catastrophic interpretation to the more realistic alternative explanation written on the Anti-Panic Flashcard.

⋛ Troubleshooting Tips ⋚

If you have trouble creating your flashcard, review the discussion of developing an alternative perspective and your Normal Anxiety Card from Exercise 6.8. Make sure you choose alternative explanations for the sensations that are the most probable and

Symptom Reappraisal

Date: _____

Instructions: Use this form to generate alternative explanations for why you're experiencing the physical or mental sensations that make you feel anxious or panicky.

Note the Physical Sensation Experienced (e.g., racing heart, breathlessness, nausea)	List Alternative Explanations for the Sensations Other than the Worst Outcome (i.e., the feared catastrophe)		Rate Belief in Each Explanation When Not Anxious (0–100)*
1.	a.		
	b.		
	c.		
2.	a.		
	b.		
	c.		
3.	a.		
	b.		
	c.		
4.	a.		
	b.		
	c.		
5.	a.		
	b.		
	c.		

*For belief ratings, 0 = absolutely no belief in the explanation, 100 = absolutely certain that this is the cause of the physical sensations.

realistic—the ones that fit the facts. If you're not sure, ask an expert like your family physician what, for example, is the most common cause of healthy people feeling they're not getting enough air. But ask only once and be satisfied with the answer.

If you're like most people with panic, you probably have no trouble believing the Anti-Panic Flashcard when calm, but when you're anxious your mind completely ignores the alternative and jumps right to the catastrophic misinterpretation of the physical sensation. So the goal of panic reappraisal is to transfer what you've learned when calm to what you think when you're anxious. You do this through PRACTICE, PRACTICE, PRACTICE!! Practice catching the catastrophic misinterpretation during anxiety episodes and correcting it with the anti-panic alternative explanation.

Decatastrophizing Panic

It takes repeated practice and evidence gathering to start the process of overriding the catastrophic misinterpretation with the alternative, benign explanation when you're anxious. Eventually you'll come to believe in the Anti-Panic Flashcard more than the catastrophic interpretation so you are using symptom reappraisal as an effective cognitive tool to reduce panic.

An old Norwegian proverb says "Experience is the best teacher, but the tuition is high." Lucia discovered this truth during the course of her cognitive therapy. The core problem for Lucia was her fear that she might have a heart attack. She became highly anxious about any tightness or pains in her chest or increase in her heart rate. Even the slightest anxiety was intolerable to her because it might lead to a panic attack. Lucia, then, was catastrophizing on many different levels. A critical element of her therapy was learning to tolerate the physical symptoms of anxiety; that is, learning to accept rather than fear tightness or pressure in her chest and increased heart rate. This was done by having Lucia complete *symptom induction exercises.*

After confirmation that she was in excellent physical health from her family physician, Lucia engaged in a series of exercises that involved intentionally causing chest muscle tension and accelerated heart rate. For example, she engaged in 2 minutes of hyperventilation followed by controlled breathing, first in the therapy session and then several times a day between sessions. This was intended to help Lucia learn to tolerate a sense of breathlessness and increased heart rate. In addition, she started a physical fitness program of aerobic exercise to gain repeated experience of heightened cardiorespiratory activity, and she started walking more quickly up flights of stairs and drinking a little extra coffee to stimulate physiological arousal. With repeated experience Lucia learned not to fear increased cardiorespiratory activity. This became an important intervention that contributed to a dramatic reduction in her panic attacks.

Symptom induction is:

> *any intentional activity that is produced to provoke an unwanted, feared physical symptom or mental/emotional state.*

Table 9.2 presents a number of symptom induction exercises used in cognitive therapy for panic. The actual exercise is described along with the primary physical sensation evoked by the experience.

There are three reasons symptom induction exercises have positive therapeutic value:

TABLE 9.2. **Examples of Symptom Induction Exercises**

Induction exercise	Provoked symptom(s)
Hyperventilate for 1–2 minutes.	Breathlessness, smothering sensation
Hold breath for 30 seconds.	Breathlessness, smothering sensation
Place tongue depressor at back of tongue for 30 seconds.	Choking sensation
Run on the spot for 1 minute.	Pounding, racing heart
Spin in a chair for approximately 1 minute.	Dizzy, faint feeling
Tense all body muscles for 1 minute.	Trembling, shaking
Breathe through narrow straw for 2 minutes.	Breathlessness, smothering sensation
Shake head rapidly from side to side for 30 seconds.	Dizzy, faint feeling
Stare continuously at yourself in the mirror for 2 minutes.	Feeling unreal, dreamy; dizzy or faint

- By generating the distressing sensation, the exercise activates your core fear and threat-related thinking so you have an opportunity to deal with it.

- It challenges your catastrophic misinterpretation that the physical sensation is dangerous by providing experiences where it does not lead to the dreaded outcome (e.g., suffocation, heart attack, seizure, full-blown panic).

- It gives you a greater sense of control over your emotional state because you're turning the physical sensation on and off.

Ultimately, the main purpose of symptom induction exercises is to provide you with numerous experiences of producing the feared physical or emotional sensation without its leading to a dreaded outcome. These exercises can provide powerful evidence that contradicts your automatic catastrophic misinterpretation. In other words, chest pressure, breathlessness, or stomach queasiness most often don't lead to heart attacks, suffocation, or vomiting but repeatedly become associated with benign outcomes.

Symptom induction can powerfully alter how you interpret the key physical or emotional sensations that make you anxious, but you have to practice it repeatedly to use it as an opportunity to reappraise your panic-related thinking.

Self-Help Exercise 9.5. Symptom Induction

Develop a schedule for engaging in symptom induction early in your cognitive therapy program. **Follow the steps below and try to engage in symptom induction daily, or at least several times a week.** Vary the exercises so you're doing a variety of activities that provoke unwanted, uncomfortable physical or emotional sensations. Use the induction exercise to practice correcting catastrophic misinterpretations of the physical sensations or other types of biased thinking about threat and danger. You can use Worksheet 6.3 to record your experiences with symptom induction as evidence that challenges anxious interpretations of the physical or emotional sensations.

Steps for Using Symptom Induction

- Step 1: Obtain medical clearance.

- Step 2: Know your core physical sensation and catastrophic misinterpretation. Focus on the primary physical, mental, or emotional sensation that makes you anxious. Write down the automatic catastrophic misinterpretation associated with the sensation from your panic log (Worksheet 9.4).

■ **Step 3: Select two or three activities that increase the unwanted sensation.** Write down a few activities that you can do that will cause an increase in the unwanted, uncomfortable sensation. You can use some of the exercises in Table 9.2 or devise your own exercises.

■ **Step 4: Begin in safety.** Make sure you begin the induction exercises in a safe, calm, and comfortable location. If you are engaged in therapy, inductions are likely to begin in your therapy sessions.

■ **Step 5: Be courageous.** Before you start, decide how long you will engage in the exercise. Don't stop when you begin to feel anxious—you're supposed to feel anxious. Keep going until you have reached the predetermined end (i.e., 2 minutes).

■ **Step 6: Take it gradually.** Begin with exercises that make you moderately anxious. Gradually increase the length of the exercise until you are completing the full exercise. For example, if a few seconds of overbreathing makes you highly anxious, start with 20 seconds and then gradually increase the duration until you are doing the full 2-minute exercise.

■ **Step 7: Reappraise the symptoms.** During the exercise, practice correcting your anxious thinking with evidence that the symptoms are benign, not dangerous. Use your Anti-Panic Flashcard and record your responses on the Symptom Reappraisal form (Worksheet 9.6).

■ **Step 8: Vary the situation.** After you've succeeded in doing symptom induction in nonanxious situations, practice producing the physical sensations in anxious or stressful situations. This is the very best way to overcome your fear of the physical symptoms of anxiety.

■ **Step 9: Practice daily and as often as possible.** It takes lots of repeated practice to benefit from symptom induction. Doing an induction exercise once or twice will not be a "game changer." The benefit comes from repetition.

⋛ Troubleshooting Tips ⋚

If you tried doing some of the symptom induction exercises and did not find them helpful, make sure you have chosen the best exercises for you—the ones that provoke your main panic-related physical sensation. If the exercise is just too overwhelming at the beginning, try a milder version and then work up to the more intense form of the exercise. To maximize their effectiveness, make sure you do the symptom induction exercises in a variety of situations that trigger your anxiety.

Confronting Fear Triggers

As you know, if you suffer from panic attacks you quickly learn which situations are most likely to trigger a panic attack and avoid these situations as much as possible. The problem is that the list of avoided situations expands over time, so many people with panic develop full-blown agoraphobia. This is why systematic exposure to avoided situations is an important component of cognitive therapy for panic disorder.

Chapter 7 discussed how to develop an exposure plan. The recommendations and monitoring forms presented in that chapter can be used to construct an exposure program that involves systematic confrontation of panic triggers. The only modification is to ensure that your exposure focuses on situations you think are high risk for triggering anxiety or panic attacks. Once again the critical elements are (1) gradually increase the difficulty level of the exposure exercises, (2) ensure that each exposure session lasts until your anxiety declines by at least half, and (3) practice correcting the automatic thoughts of threat and danger that occur during exposure. Use your exposure sessions to practice training your attention on the safety aspects of situations (e.g., "What is the evidence that I'm actually safe standing here in the mall even though I'm feeling incredibly anxious?") and learning to tolerate, even accept, the state of feeling anxious. Remind yourself of the *AWARE* strategy presented in Chapter 7, page 142.

Self-Help Exercise 9.6.
Exposure for Panic

Construct a hierarchy of panic-related triggers that starts with moderately distressing situations that you usually avoid and moves up to panic-inducing situations you always avoid. Begin with the moderately distressing situations and engage in repeated situational exposure several times a week. Continue exposing yourself to a situation until you can do it with half as much anxiety as when you began. Then move on to the next situation in your hierarchy. Exposure is complete when you no longer avoid the situations in your hierarchy.

> ≳ **Troubleshooting Tips** ≲
>
> If you have difficulty following an exposure plan, review Chapter 7 and the work you completed in that chapter. This will help you remember strategies you can use to overcome barriers to exposure.

If agoraphobic avoidance is prominent in your panic disorder, exposure will play a much bigger part in your treatment strategy. Reduction in avoidance through exposure is vital to reducing the frequency and severity of full-blown and limited-symptom panic attacks.

CHAPTER SUMMARY

■ Panic attacks are characterized as a sudden onset of intense fear or discomfort involving a number of physical and emotional sensations.

■ Heightened anxiety sensitivity, or fear of fear, is a major contributor to the persistence of panic that is targeted in cognitive therapy.

■ The key elements in the cognitive basis of panic are (1) heightened awareness and monitoring of certain physical or emotional sensations, (2) automatic catastrophic misinterpretation of these sensations, (3) an inability to reevaluate and correct the misinterpretation, and (4) reliance on avoidance and safety-seeking behaviors to "control" panic.

■ Cognitive therapy begins with the construction of your panic profile that will guide your intervention program.

■ Weekly panic logs (Worksheet 9.4) are kept throughout the course of treatment to collect relevant information and evaluate the effectiveness of your intervention.

■ Panic symptom reappraisal and development of an Anti-Panic Flashcard are the central elements of cognitive therapy for panic. Reduction in panic attacks can occur only when you learn to correct the automatic catastrophic misinterpretation of physical or emotional symptoms.

■ Symptom induction exercises are used to activate anxious thinking (i.e., excessive threatening thoughts and misinterpretations) so that you learn to correct your catastrophic misinterpretations and tolerate heightened anxiety states.

■ Systematic exposure to panic triggers is an important component of a cognitive therapy program when panic is associated with extensive avoidance of situations and overreliance on maladaptive safety-seeking behaviors to control anxiety.

10

Conquering Social Fear

This chapter is especially relevant for you if:

- Your anxiety occurs almost exclusively when you're around people and remains a problem even though you've worked through the Anxiety Work Plan you created in Chapter 8.

- You have a lot of anticipatory anxiety about social interactions that was not addressed by your Anxiety Work Plan.

- You still find yourself worrying about how you acted or what you said to others, and this makes you feel terribly anxious.

- You still avoid social situations even though you've made some progress on your anxiety.

- You continue to be overly concerned about what people think of you.

Martin was painfully shy, or at least that's how he'd always thought of himself. Even as a child he had always felt nervous, especially around other kids. He remembers feeling quite lonely then, with only one close friend and living in fear that attention would be drawn to him in the classroom. Now, 33, single, and working for a software developer, he continues to feel alone and isolated. A few years ago he had to move several hours away from his family for a new job, and the adjustment has been difficult. In the last 6 months he's started to feel really down, losing interest in things he once enjoyed, feeling like he has no energy, and sleeping poorly. His doctor said he was depressed and started him on antidepressants, which made him feel a little better, but a deep sense of loneliness, boredom, and dissatisfaction lingers.

Martin kept to himself at work. At first coworkers tried to include him in conversation and invited him for drinks after work. But Martin always turned them down. He felt tense, awkward, and self-conscious around others and didn't seem to know how to carry on a casual conversation. When he got anxious, his face flushed, he started to tremble, his heart raced, he felt hot and sweaty, and he felt like he couldn't breathe properly. He was convinced other people noticed his anxiety and were thinking "What's wrong with him?" and "What's he so nervous about?" and "Is he mentally ill?" In this state of intense anxiety, Martin was convinced other people were staring at him and conjuring up all sorts of negative conclusions about the way he acted, and the minute they paid attention to him his self-consciousness increased.

On occasion when he tried to say something, the words didn't come out right and he was left feeling deeply ashamed and embarrassed. Sometimes he would mentally rehearse what to say to people, but this seemed to make matters worse because when uttered out loud it came across as canned and insincere. If he was told about a meeting scheduled at work, Martin's anxiety escalated the closer he got to the event until the anticipatory anxiety was unbearable. He might spend a couple of sleepless nights worrying about how he could cope with any upcoming social occasion. Although he would feel some relief afterward, it was always short-lived because he would start mentally rehashing the event and what people might have thought of him. This tendency to replay past social interactions over and over—what we call *postevent rumination*—would often cause him to conclude that he had embarrassed himself once again, which only cemented his conviction that he was hopeless around other people.

Martin's main strategy for coping with his intense social anxiety was *avoidance*. He avoided a variety of interpersonal situations, such as making appointments, attending social gatherings or having a friend over for dinner, starting conversations and expressing opinions, going on dates, and answering the phone, as well as numerous performance situations, like speaking at meetings, eating/drinking in public, shopping in a busy store, walking in front of a group of people, and performing before an audience. If he couldn't avoid a social situation, Martin would say as little as possible and leave as soon as he could. He found his anxiety was a little better if he had a few drinks and kept a tranquilizer handy in case he started to have a panic attack.

Martin suffers from *social phobia* (or social anxiety disorder), one of the most common forms of anxiety disorder, which afflicts an estimated 15 million American adults (6.8%) in a given year.[39] This condition often begins in childhood or early adolescence, and it can take a chronic course that lasts for decades. Social phobia can cause a lifetime of disappointment, loneliness, and distress and is often associated with other disorders like major depression, generalized anxiety, and alcohol use disorders.[5] Milder forms of social anxiety are even more common in the general population, and heightened anxiety in social situations is a frequent complaint in a variety of anxiety disorders. Despite making progress on your anxiety in the earlier chapters, you may be feeling that social anxiety, even though a minor part of your anxiety problem, was not addressed adequately. In this chapter we focus on social anxiety generally and discuss interventions you can use that are specifically designed to reduce heightened social and evaluative anxiety.

What Will People Think?

We all care what others think of us. It's perfectly natural as human beings to want to be liked by others, to receive their approval, acceptance, and maybe even their admiration. Compliments, praise, and positive feedback from significant people in our lives make us feel great; criticism, rejection, disapproval, and negative feedback feel terrible. Feeling embarrassed is one of the most uncomfortable, if not traumatic, emotions we all feel, so of course we try our best to avoid making a negative impression. Let's face it, we all like to fit in, to feel like we're accepted and one of the crowd.

So it's perfectly normal to feel somewhat nervous and tense when we find ourselves in an unfamiliar social situation or have to introduce ourselves, carry on conversations, or give our opinion—all while appearing relaxed, confident, and even engaging or witty. Everyone thinks at times "How am I doing?", "I wonder what they think of me?", "I hope I didn't say something stupid," "I really feel like a fish out of water," or "I can't wait to get out of here." We look for indications from others that we're doing okay, that we fit in; and we may feel uneasy, even embarrassed, if we pick up that others are bored, uninterested, or, worse, annoyed with us. After leaving these awkward social interactions, we rehash the night's events in our minds—how we "performed," other people's reactions to us—trying to come to some conclusion on the question "Did I make a fool of myself?"

If you have social anxiety, everything we just described probably feels magnified a thousand times. Maybe you feel paralyzed by fear in social situations, living in dread of making a negative impression. The possibility of embarrassing yourself may have become a full-blown catastrophe that you can't risk. You're so convinced that you look awkward and inept that you start monitoring your every verbal utterance and gesture in an effort to make a good impression. But over time you seem to be losing the battle: the harder you try to fit in, the worse the perceived outcome. You're sure you've embarrassed yourself, so you look back at social interactions with shame, remembering them as the worst experiences in your life. Eventually you decide you can't put yourself through such torture anymore; better to avoid others as much as possible than endure such humiliation. And so you start isolating yourself, withdrawing behind walls of self-protection, barricading yourself from the rest of humanity. But this comes at a great cost; you often feel alone, with a profound sense of dissatisfaction and reduced quality of life. The other great cost is that you become less practiced in the "arts of social discourse" and so feel more and more awkward in social situations. You're caught in a vicious cycle that seems impossible to escape!

Three Core Elements of Social Anxiety

There are three core components of intense social anxiety, and each is specifically targeted in cognitive therapy for social phobia.

1. *Fear of negative evaluation*—the fear of being judged negatively by others and incurring their scorn and disdain; fear that others will think you're stupid, weak, inept, maybe even crazy.

2. *Heightened self-focus*—being intensely focused on your social performance, imagining how you're coming across to others to the point where you can barely hear what people are saying. Paradoxically, the more you try to control and evaluate every utterance, facial expression, and gesture, the more awkward you become in your social interactions.

3. *Extensive avoidance*—avoiding people as much as possible and escaping at the earliest opportunity when forced into social situations.

Martin was gripped with fear that others would notice his anxiety in social situations. He was convinced they would notice his flushed face, trembling hands, and halting speech and then wonder what was wrong with him. He told himself they were probably thinking, "Poor guy—he looks so anxious," "What a weak, pathetic person who can't even relate to other people," or "He probably has some severe mental illness." This highly negative view made him so self-conscious that his anxiety increased—but it also made his concern about his lack of conversational skills actually come true as it made it even harder for him to listen and concentrate on what people were saying to him. In the end the anxiety was so great that Martin would leave these social functions as soon as possible. Escape brought him instant, unbelievable relief. Every time, he would vow never to put himself through such torture again.

Cognitive therapy for social anxiety targets the three core elements in social evaluative anxiety: excessive fear of negative evaluations, heightened self-focus, and extensive avoidance.

People with social anxiety not only fear the negative evaluation of others but also often have high standards of social performance—like they should be witty and entertaining or should feel perfectly relaxed, comfortable, and confident. Of course, setting standards so high that they're impossible to reach only increases anxiety and reinforces the conviction that "I just can't handle social situations." What is your social ideal—and what negative evaluation do you dread? Record both on Worksheet 10.1.

When Does Social Anxiety Become a Problem?

In one survey 40% of people considered themselves chronically shy,[40] and in another general population study 7.5% of adults had significant symptoms of social anxiety.[41] If you happen to find yourself at one of those uncomfortable cocktail parties where you hardly know anyone, look around you. If there are 50 people at this party, there is a good chance that at least 20 of them are feeling at least some discom-

My Ideal Impression
versus Feared Negative Evaluation by Others

Instructions: In the space below, write a brief description of the ideal impression you would like to make on others: What is the most positive opinion people could have about you? How would you like people to see you? What type of impression would you like to make on people (e.g., for them to think of you as very friendly, witty, intelligent, relaxed, outgoing)?

My Most Positive Impression

_____

_____

_____

_____

_____

Instructions: In the space below, write a brief description of the most negative impression you could make on others. What would be the most negative opinion others could have about you? What is your most feared negative evaluation (e.g., that you are stupid, a loner, pathetic, weak, insecure, unstable)?

_____

_____

_____

_____

_____

It's common to feel some anxiety and discomfort in unfamiliar social settings or when we're being watched by others, like when making a speech or performing in front of people. If your social anxiety is more extreme, the interventions in this chapter can be used to turn down your social anxiety to a more manageable level.

fort and maybe five people are feeling fairly intense levels of anxiety. But if social anxiety is a significant problem for you, especially if it hasn't been reduced by your work in Chapters 1–8 of this book, it's probably worth considering spending some time on the additional exercises in this chapter. If several of the questions on Worksheet 10.2 apply to you, the cognitive therapy strategies discussed in this chapter will be particularly relevant for you because they are designed for people with moderate to severe social anxiety.

The Socially Anxious Mind

Like other anxiety conditions, social anxiety operates as a vicious cycle. You anticipate social encounters with some degree of trepidation, then you find yourself in the social situation experiencing unhelpful thoughts and actions that drive up your anxiety, and then afterward you rehash and brood over the social encounter, which only exaggerates the dread with which you anticipate the next social interaction. The cognitive model, with its three phases, is depicted in the diagram on page 199.

1. Anticipatory Phase

Although social interactions can occur spontaneously and unexpectedly (such as when you run into a work colleague while shopping), most often we know about meetings, interviews, and parties well in advance. This means we have lots of time to think about, ponder, and even worry about the upcoming social event. This is called the *anticipatory phase*. Depending on the type of future social event, anxiety can build dramatically during a period of anticipation. For example, if your supervisor has asked you to give a brief presentation at this Friday's department meeting, anticipatory anxiety will be much greater than if you simply have to attend. Many of our clients have said that their anxiety is often more intense during anticipation than when they are actually exposed to the event. Two things will influence the degree of anticipatory anxiety you experience:

1. *How far ahead the event is:* The closer you get to a dreaded social event, the more intense your anxiety because anxiety builds over the anticipatory phase.

2. *Exaggerated thinking about threat:* Catastrophizing about the social event, thinking that you'll probably embarrass or humiliate yourself, or maybe have

Social Anxiety Checklist

Instructions: Read each question and determine whether the item is *mostly relevant* to your current functioning in social situations. If you answered "yes" to more than five or six questions, then social anxiety is probably a significant issue for you.

Questions	Yes	No
1. Do you almost always feel quite anxious in a variety of social situations that you encounter on a daily basis?		
2. Do you often feel apprehensive or worried about upcoming social events?		
3. Do you avoid or make excuses to get out of social obligations?		
4. When you can't avoid a social encounter, do you try to leave as soon as possible?		
5. Do you tend to assume you are making a poor impression on people or that they are judging you in a negative manner (e.g., thinking you are stupid, incompetent, disturbed)?		
6. Are you intensely afraid of saying something embarrassing or humiliating when talking to others?		
7. Do you try hard not to appear anxious in social situations?		
8. When you are around other people, do you try to say as little as possible to avoid drawing attention to yourself?		
9. In social situations, are you quite preoccupied with your performance, tending to "overanalyze" how you are coming across to other people?		
10. Do you rely on various coping strategies to reduce your anxiety around others, such as avoiding eye contact, rehearsing what you say before speaking, or taking deep breaths?		
11. Has social anxiety held you back in your occupation, family relations, leisure activities, or friendships?		
12. After a social interaction, do you often go over and over in your mind what you said or how you came across to other people?		
13. Do you seem to have a particularly good memory for difficult or embarrassing past social encounters?		
14. Do you often feel like you don't know what to say to other people?		
15. Do you believe you are particularly incompetent or inept around other people?		
16. Is embarrassing yourself in front of others just about the worst thing you can imagine?		
17. Do you have problems being assertive or stating your opinion?		
18. Would people who know you best say you are a shy or anxious person?		
19. Do you feel like everyone is looking at you in social situations?		
20. Do you think you are more anxious in social situations than most people?		
21. Have you been socially anxious or inhibited most of your life?		
22. Have you tried to overcome social anxiety but had only limited success in beating it?		

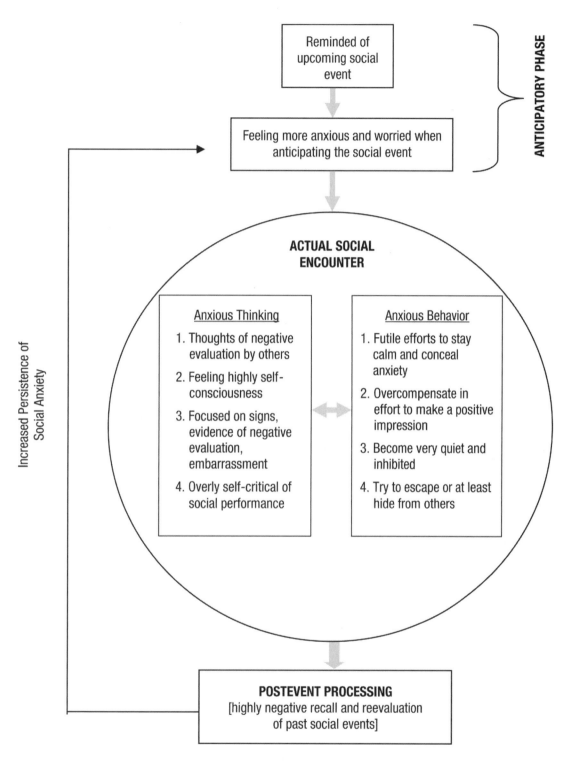

The cognitive model of social anxiety.

a panic attack, and predicting that you'll perform badly based on memories of past social events, will also drive up your anxiety level.

The problem with anticipatory anxiety is that it sets the stage for feeling intense anxiety even before you encounter the social situation. *It makes you feel defeated before you even get started!* Martin suffered intense anticipatory anxiety whenever he had to interact with unfamiliar people. One morning last week a work colleague popped into Martin's office and invited him to lunch with a few people in the office and one of the new hires in the department. Martin felt he couldn't refuse but then worried all morning about the lunch: "What would I say? I'm so bad at chit-chat!" "What if I get really nervous and self-conscious?" "Will others notice my anxiety and wonder what's wrong with me?" "Last time I went out with people at work, I felt like such a dork, just sitting there with nothing to say while everyone else was talking and laughing." Martin hadn't been able to face anyone at work for several days after that incident without feeling intensely embarrassed. Now his anxious thinking was so bad that he could hardly work. By lunchtime he was feeling intensely anxious.

> We can literally whip ourselves into a heightened state of anxiety even before a social event occurs. Cognitive therapy reduces anticipatory anxiety by modifying anxiety-inducing expectations.

2. Social Exposure Phase

As you can see in the diagram "The Cognitive Model of Social Anxiety," once you're actually in a social situation, all kinds of anxious thoughts and behaviors kick in.

Negative Social Beliefs

One of the first things that's likely to happen when you enter an interpersonal situation is that underlying negative beliefs about yourself and other people are activated. Some beliefs that are common in social anxiety are listed in Table 10.1. If any of these beliefs are relevant for you, underline them—they'll become an important focus of your cognitive therapy work plan.

Several of Martin's beliefs increased his anxiety when around other people. He was convinced he was very dull and boring but felt like he should strive to be engaging and entertaining and appear relaxed and confident. Therefore it seemed critical to him to conceal his anxiety as much as possible—not only would others judge him harshly if they noticed he was nervous, but feeling embarrassed seemed like just about the worst thing that could happen to him. "Better to avoid people as much as possible than to risk embarrassment or humiliation," Martin believed.

TABLE 10.1. **Beliefs That Characterize Social Anxiety**

Type of belief	Examples of specific beliefs
Beliefs about the self	• "I'm boring, unfriendly, and uninteresting to others." • "People don't tend to like me." • "I'm socially awkward; I don't fit in."
Beliefs about others	• "People tend to be highly critical." • "In social situations people are always judging me, scrutinizing other people, looking for their flaws and weaknesses."
Beliefs about disapproval	• "It's awful when people disapprove of me." • "It would be horrible if others thought I was weak or incompetent." • "It is a personal catastrophe to embarrass oneself in front of others." • "People don't want to include me; they would like to exclude me from their social events."
Beliefs about performance	• "It's important not to show any signs of weakness or loss of control around others." • "I must appear confident and interpersonally competent in all my social interactions." • "I must always sound intelligent, come across as interesting, or be entertaining around other people."
Beliefs about anxiety	• "Anxiety is a sign of weakness and loss of control." • "It is important not to show any signs of anxiety around others." • "If people see that I'm blushing, perspiring, shaking, etc., they will wonder what's wrong with me." • "If I'm anxious, I won't be able to function in this social situation." • "I can't stand feeling anxious around people."

Reprinted with permission from *Cognitive Therapy of Anxiety Disorders* by David A. Clark and Aaron T. Beck (p. 350). Copyright 2010 by The Guilford Press.

Thoughts about Being Evaluated Negatively

If you're socially anxious, you automatically think that other people are noticing your anxiety and making negative judgments about your behavior and wondering what's wrong with you. You might imagine that other people are thinking: "What's wrong with her?" "Why is she so anxious?" "She must be emotionally disturbed." "That was a stupid thing to say." "She is so incompetent, I wish she would just keep quiet or disappear." Like other anxious thoughts, these negative evaluative cognitions are automatic and are quite convincing during states of heightened anxiety. And once you start thinking this way, you probably find it hard to concentrate on anything other than the bad impression you're making. It's as if social anxiety leaves you with a one-track mind: *people are thinking poorly of me.*

Biased Attention

When we're anxious in a social situation, our attention also becomes distorted. First we become entirely self-focused. Experimental research has shown that socially anxious individuals engage in excessive self-monitoring and negatively misinterpret their physical and emotional sensations in a manner that actually increases their anxiety.[5] You might become preoccupied with whether your face looks flushed, whether your hands are trembling, whether your conversation makes sense, whether your speech flows or is halting and awkward. Of course this heightened self-consciousness has a negative effect:

- It magnifies anxiety symptoms and a sense of losing control.

- It causes you to be so entirely self-focused you can't properly pay attention to how other people are responding to you.

- It impairs your ability to perform socially.

Second, when you're socially anxious your attention becomes narrowly focused on internal and external signs of threat, embarrassment, and negative evaluation. Say you're nervously trying to make a comment. Your attention becomes fixed on the person checking her smartphone or glancing in the other direction. Immediately you interpret these cues as a sign of boredom and disinterest in you. When you're already feeling anxious, your attention becomes highly selective and you tend to lock on to any facial expression, behavior, or gesture that could suggest a negative evaluation and fail to notice indicators that people are supportive or interested in you. We do the same with our internal experience, paying attention to flushed sensations that we interpret as indicating overt anxiety but ignoring that our speech is coherent and flows reasonably well. In cognitive therapy we teach people how to correct their biased attention so they can lower their social anxiety rather than fuel it.

Self-Critical Thoughts

When you're intensely focused on your own performance, you're likely to quickly jump to the conclusion that you're making a poor impression or actually experiencing public humiliation. You probably engage in a running commentary on your social performance, concluding that you're failing miserably. Martin was especially self-conscious about whether he was blushing while talking to others. He became acutely aware of feeling hot or flushed, and the first signs that he was blushing would distract him from the conversation at hand. He assumed the blushing was more noticeable and distracting to others than it was and that it was making his ability to converse less coherent and more awkward. He quickly assumed that he was making a horrible impression and really embarrassing himself in front of others.

Behaviors Intended to Reduce or Conceal Anxiety

You may have tried a number of measures to reduce your anxiety or at least to conceal it from others. Maybe you avoid eye contact, tense your arms or legs to control shaking, wear excessive clothing to conceal sweating, wear heavy makeup to hide blushing, or memorize what to say at social gatherings as Martin tried to do.[42] Unfortunately, some of these safety behaviors actually draw more attention to you rather than less. One woman believed that exaggerated controlled breathing calmed her down, but her breathing was so loud and labored that it could be heard several feet away, possibly drawing the attention of others, who might have wondered whether she was having an asthma attack or some other medical emergency.

> Cognitive therapy focuses intensely on correcting the social anxiety mind-set—the assumption that you're being evaluated negatively, the inclination to hold a running commentary on your own performance and how unsatisfactory it is, and the conclusion that you've embarrassed yourself. These corrections make you less anxious and enable you to behave more effectively in social situations.

Overdoing It

In an effort to overcome perceived social skills deficits and make a positive impression, have you ever caught yourself overcompensating? You might have occasionally tried so hard to be funny, intelligent, or friendly that you inadvertently made an unfavorable impression. When Martin realized he tended to look down when talking to others, he tried to correct the habit by looking right at them but ended up staring so hard that other people became uncomfortable.

> Trying hard to stay calm, attempting to conceal anxiety, trying to compensate for social awkwardness, and being generally inhibited can all lead to the actual thing that you fear most—negative evaluation and embarrassment. Cognitive therapy focuses on modifying these coping responses so that your interpersonal behavior reduces rather than intensifies anxiety.

Social Inhibition and Escape

Anticipating embarrassment naturally makes you inhibited around others. You may feel like you seem stiff or rigid. Perhaps you stammer or struggle to find the right word to express your thoughts. If you've had this experience, you know it's as if the very thing you fear most is actually happening to you. When it does, it's no wonder you have the urge to escape. Because everything he tried to say seemed to come out wrong, Martin was determined to stick by himself or at least say as little as possible when he couldn't avoid a social encounter.

3. Postevent Processing Phase

In many respects social anxiety is "the gift that keeps on giving." Although you may experience relief after leaving an anxiety-arousing social situation, the reprieve is usually short lived. Soon you find yourself rehashing and overanalyzing a social encounter— "How did I perform?" and "Did I say something stupid, rude, or embarrassing?"— and trying to recall what people said to determine whether you made a good or bad impression. But this postmortem tends to be very selective: you keep asking yourself whether the social encounter was a humiliating disaster, and the more you ruminate on that question, the more evidence you tend to unearth to answer it with a "yes." This postevent processing could last hours or even several days, depending on the importance of the event. Most of the rehashing goes on in your own mind, but sometimes you might ask repeatedly for feedback from close friends or family. Typically with social anxiety, no matter what others say to the contrary, you end up convinced that "Yes, it was a terrible experience, I completely embarrassed myself, and everyone probably thinks I'm a total jerk." The end result? Your social anxiety is reinforced and therefore persists.

> It is common in social anxiety to "relive" what you perceive as past embarrassing social encounters in a selective and highly biased way that leads to an exaggerated perception of shame and embarrassment. Since this postevent processing is a key contributor to social anxiety, it becomes an important target for change in cognitive therapy.

Postevent processing was a significant problem in Martin's social anxiety. He could spend days reanalyzing what he said in a conversation and how the other person responded. The more he thought about it, the more convinced he became that his anxiety was on full display and that his conversation was so incoherent that it had left the other person perplexed, convinced that Martin must be emotionally disturbed. In some cases he found himself trying to avoid this person at work and feeling embarrassed every time he ran into him. On occasion Martin even thought that maybe the work colleague was telling others about the strange conversation he had had with him.

Your Social Anxiety Profile

The first step in overcoming social anxiety is to develop a thorough understanding of the problem. Once you understand how you are making yourself excessively anxious in social situations, you'll be able to make important changes that will eventually reduce your anxiety level. The following steps, based on the cognitive model on page 199, will enable you to build a profile of your social anxiety.

Step 1: Create a Hierarchy of Situations and Goals

Using the Exposure Hierarchy form from Chapter 7 (Worksheet 7.3), write down approximately 20 social situations that make you feel anxious. Make sure you capture a full range of social activities, from ones that cause you mild discomfort to those that cause severe anxiety. Also choose some situations that occur daily, many that occur weekly, and only a couple that occur less frequently. For example, giving a speech might be the most anxiety-provoking situation you can imagine, but unless your job requires public speaking, you may rarely have an opportunity to give a speech and so should exclude this from your hierarchy. After you've developed your list of situations, arrange them hierarchically from least to most anxiety provoking. We will be returning to these situations later in the chapter.

Before starting to work on your social anxiety, it's important to be clear on your goals for change. What would you like to achieve from this chapter? How would you like to feel and act in social situations? How would you like to socialize? Taking some of the key social situations listed in your hierarchy, briefly describe how you would like to act and feel in these situations using Worksheet 10.3. These will become the specific goals for your therapy program.

Step 2: Rate Your Anticipatory Anxiety

Think back to some recent experiences with social anxiety (or refer to what you will record on Worksheet 10.5 on page 209) and use Worksheet 10.4 to record your level of anxiety in the hours, days, or maybe even weeks prior to the event. On that form you should also fill in whether the anxiety got worse as the event neared and what you were thinking about the approaching event—what you worried might happen, how others might respond to you or how you might feel and act, how well you envisioned dealing with the situation, and whether you were thinking about similar past events and whether the same perceived embarrassment would occur again this time around.

Step 3: Identify Your Anxious Thinking in Social Encounters

How you think about yourself, other people, and your anxiety will determine whether you experience mild or severe anxiety. So it's important to discover your thought patterns during actual social encounters.

Goals for Personal Social Change

Instructions: Select four or five social situations from your hierarchy that cause moderate to severe anxiety and yet are critical to your quality of life. Write these in the left-hand column and then use the right-hand column to record how you would like to feel, act, and think in those situations if you had only minimal anxiety. What would be a *realistic goal* for your level of performance or functioning in these situations? These will become your therapy goals and can be used to judge how well you are progressing with your cognitive therapy program.

Social Situation	Description of Social Performance Goal
1.	1.
2.	2.
3.	3.
4.	4.
5.	5.

Analysis of Your Anticipatory Social Anxiety

Situation Where Anticipatory Anxiety Occurred Also note anything that triggered your anticipatory anxiety.	Severity of Anxiety (0–100) and Its Duration (hours, days, weeks, etc.)	Anticipated Threat What are you thinking might happen? What's the worst possible outcome you anticipate might happen?	Recalled Past Memories Are you recalling similar past social events that ended in high anxiety or embarrassment?

Self-Help Exercise 10.1.
Recording Your Social Interactions

Keep a record of your social interactions for the duration of your cognitive therapy program using the Monitoring Your Social Anxiety form (Worksheet 10.5), completing the form right after a social event that provoked your anxiety. Recording your anxious social encounters will reveal that your social anxiety varies across situations. By keeping a self-monitoring sheet you'll train yourself to identify ways of thinking and coping that make your anxiety worse as well as helpful responses that reduce anxiety.

To fill out the form, ask yourself these questions:

■ *Negative evaluation thoughts:* "What was I afraid other people in that social situation might think about me?" "What type of negative opinion or judgment might they form about me?" "What is the worst that people might think about me?" "What was I thinking that other people thought about me?"

■ *Biased attention to social threat cues:* "What did I notice in other people that made me more anxious (e.g., a certain facial expression, behavior, verbal response)?" "What was capturing my attention in the social situation (e.g., the way a certain person looked at me)?"

■ *Heightened self-focus:* "Was I overly self-conscious?" "What specific physical sensations, thoughts, or behavior became the focus of my attention?" "What was I most self-conscious about in this social situation?"

■ *Negative self-evaluation:* "Was I overanalyzing myself?" "What was I thinking about my performance, the impression I was making on others, in this social interaction?"

■ *Beliefs about concealing anxiety:* "Was I trying to conceal my anxiety from others?" "Was there a particular anxious symptom I was most concerned about hiding from others (e.g., that I was blushing, sweating, trembling)?" "Did I think I was successfully concealing my anxiety?"

Monitoring Your Social Anxiety

Dates: from: _____ to: _____

Instructions: Use the following form to record your daily experiences with anxious or distressing social situations that may involve some performance on your part, an evaluation by others, and/or interpersonal interactions. It is important to complete this form as soon after the social event as possible to maintain its accuracy.

Date	Describe Difficult or Anxious Social Situation What happened, who was involved, where, what was your role?	Rate Level of Anticipatory Anxiety (0–100)	Rate Level of Anxiety during Event Occurrence (0–100)	Main Anxious Thoughts during Social Encounter (i.e., negative thoughts about others' evaluation, self-critical thoughts, catastrophizing)	Rate Level of Postevent Anxiety and Embarrassment (0–100)

Note. Rate level of anxiety on a scale from 0 ("no anxiety") to 50 ("moderately intense") to 100 ("extreme, panic level"). Whenever a panic attack is experienced in the anticipation, or exposure, phase, record with initials PA. (If unsure, see Chapter 9, page 166, for definition of panic attack.) In last column, also rate level of embarrassment that remains associated with the situation from 0 ("none") to 100 ("the most embarrassing, humiliating experience in my life").

Step 4: Identify Your Automatic Coping When Socially Anxious

A review of Worksheet 10.5 will reveal how you were thinking in the social situation that may have heightened your anxiety. On a blank sheet of paper, write down some of the ways you tend to respond when you are in anxiety-provoking social situations by focusing on the following areas:

- *Safety behaviors:* "How do I try to conceal my anxiety or appear that I am in control (avoid eye contact, drink lots of water, rehearse everything I will say before I say it, etc.)?" "How do I try to lower my anxiety level in social situations (e.g., take deep breaths, avoid people, have a few drinks)?"

- *Failed impression management:* "Do I act in a certain way to try to make a favorable impression on others? If so, how successful are these attempts? For example, do I talk too much about myself, or do I smile and nod too much in an effort to make a good impression?"

- *Inhibited behavior:* "Do I act in an overly inhibited or awkward manner in interpersonal situations?" "Is there anything I tend to do that is particularly embarrassing (e.g., stutter, have difficulty finding the right word, appear tongue-tied)?"

- *Escape or avoid:* "Do I tend to end up avoiding people?" "Do I say very little or leave a situation early?" "Where do I position myself in a social gathering to draw as little attention as possible?"

Step 5: Analyze Your Postevent Processing

The final component of your social anxiety profile focuses on the time period after a social experience. It's important to determine the nature and extent of your rumination over past social experiences. Table 10.2 presents a series of questions to ask yourself about the role of postevent processing in your social anxiety. These are organized around the critical aspects of postevent rumination about past social experiences. You should write down your answers to these questions, writing out a description of your postevent worry about your social experiences. The important question to answer is: *How are you thinking back on past social experiences that convinces you of embarrassment, humiliation, or shame?*

> A profile of your personal social anxiety will act as your guide through therapy and indicate what aspects of your social anxiety need to be targeted for change in the three stages of social anxiety: anticipation, social encounter, and postevent processing.

TABLE 10.2. **Probing Postevent Rumination over Past Social Experiences**

Elements	Probing questions
Reevaluating a recent social experience	• "Why am I more convinced now that people were judging me negatively?" • "What am I thinking about how I behaved or what I said that caused a negative impression on others?" • "What am I thinking happened that convinces me I embarrassed or humiliated myself?" • "The more I think about it, is the consequence of the social experience getting worse? If so, how? What am I thinking about that convinces me the experience was so awful?" • "How do I think I failed in this social interaction?" • "Looking back, how intolerable was the anxiety? Could I face a similar experience again?"
Past memories of difficult social experiences	• "Am I thinking back to past social experiences that were particularly embarrassing or when I felt especially anxious? If so, which particular events do I keep recalling?" • "What particular aspects of these memories do I focus on? Was it how people responded, how I acted, or how awful I felt?" • "What has been the longer-term consequence of these past embarrassing experiences?" • "When I recall these past events, can I imagine them, or am I thinking about the event?"

Ruminative themes	• "When I am thinking back on a social encounter, I tend to analyze over and over:
	  • How anxious I felt.
	  • Whether I was inappropriate, rude, or insulting.
	  • Whether others could tell how anxious I felt.
	  • How I was so incompetent, boring, socially awkward.
	  • How I was ignored by others and felt their disapproval.
	  • Examples of critical remarks made by others."

Transforming Negative Anticipatory Thoughts

Learning to correct the negative thoughts and beliefs that characterize the core fear in social anxiety is at the center of cognitive therapy. The cognitive strategies described in Chapter 6 can be applied to the social situations that make you anxious, and they'll be most helpful in the anticipatory and postevent processing phases. Once you have learned to correct your anxious thinking during these phases, you can work on applying these strategies in the actual social situations.

How we think about an approaching social event determines whether we feel intense or mild anticipatory anxiety. Catastrophizing about a future social situation will only make matters worse. This type of exaggerated thinking about social threat causes intense anxiety and will make you feel defeated even before you begin. So correcting this thought process is a key to reducing anticipatory anxiety and building self-confidence in social situations.

Start by identifying three social events that make you feel moderately anxious. In the space below, write down an anxiety-provoking social event that will occur in the next day or two, then an event that will occur in the next week, and finally an event that may be several weeks away but is already causing you some anxiety. (Consult Worksheet 10.4 for ideas for relevant social situations.)

Immediate social situation: _____

_____

Social situation next week: _____

_____

Distant social situation: _____

_____

Next take the immediate social situation and identify your most anxious thinking about this situation using the Threat Assessment Diary from Chapter 6 (Worksheet 6.2). Try to answer the following questions about your anticipatory thinking:

- "What do I think is the worst possible outcome in this situation?"

- "What do I think is the worst possible way that I will feel or behave in this situation?"

- "What is the catastrophe, the social threat, that I fear will occur?"

- "What am I telling myself about the probability and severity of this bad outcome?"

- "Am I telling myself other people will think badly of me, that I won't be able to cope with the situation, that I will experience unbearable anxiety?"

Martin's immediate social event was a department meeting at the end of the week in which he had to give a short presentation. For several days his anxiety about this event had been building. His anticipatory anxious cognitions involved thinking everyone would be looking at him and would notice he was blushing, that they'd be thinking, "Poor Martin—he gets so anxious; he has a real problem," and that he'd probably start stuttering, lose his place, and feel extreme embarrassment. He recalled the last time he tried to give a presentation and how he felt so embarrassed at work for days after the event.

Next evaluate your anxious anticipatory thoughts using the Gathering Evidence form in Chapter 6 (Worksheet 6.3). Is there any evidence that your thinking is exaggerated? Will the anxiety really be that intolerable? Will others really think as badly about you as you anticipate? Will you embarrass yourself as much as you think? Will the event be as "life altering" as you imagine? Are you exaggerating the significance of the event, that it really is all about you, and that it will forever change people's opinion of you? You can also use Worksheet 6.4 to evaluate the short- and long-term consequences associated with feeling intense anxiety in the immediate social event. Are you exaggerating the importance and consequences of the social event?

Martin used Worksheets 6.3 and 6.4 to realize he was exaggerating the degree of social threat and importance of the department meeting. Yes, he would feel anxious, but he could get through it. Others were making presentations, so the meeting was not all about him. His coworkers knew he had public speaking anxiety, and even if his talk was a little rough, they would probably forget about it within hours or a few days. His past experiences of social anxiety had had absolutely no lasting impact on how they related to him. His anxiety was clearly a lot less significant to them than he was thinking.

After evaluating your anticipatory thinking, use the Alternative Interpretations form (Worksheet 6.5) to construct a more balanced, realistic, alternative way to think about the social event. Worksheet 6.5 allows you to generate the worst-case outcome (e.g., "I'll humiliate myself and people will think I'm totally incompetent"), the most desired outcome (e.g., "I'll feel completely relaxed and confident, and I'll impress people"), and the most probable, realistic outcome (e.g., "I'll be moderately anxious, get through it okay, and people will quickly forget about it"). You should write down evidence for each of these perspectives to determine which is most likely to occur.

The final step in transforming how you think about the most immediate social event involves creating a revised Normal Anxiety Card (see Step 8 in Chapter 6). How should you think about the approaching social event? Martin's normalization card for the Friday department meeting looked like this:

I have to give a 10-minute presentation on the new mobile device synchronization program we are introducing to company employees. I will feel moderately anxious making this presentation. I will get red in the face, I'll probably feel hot, and I may stumble over some of my words. It won't be the best presentation at the meeting. However, I will be able to communicate the main points of my presentation. I notice other people seem to get anxious when they present and yet life goes on. My public speaking performance matters a lot less to my coworkers than I think. They all know I get anxious when I make presentations, and it hasn't changed how they relate to me. In the past I've never done anything embarrassing or inappropriate other than feel intense anxiety. I can write out what I am going to say, practice making the speech, and actually learn to deliver it even when feeling intense anxiety. If I'm asked a question I can't answer, I can simply write it down and say I'll get back to the person with the answer later. So the bottom line is that I will feel anxious but I will be able to make the presentation. It's an event that will have no lasting impact. It's not going to alter what my coworkers already think about me.

On the more positive side, it gives me an opportunity to practice and improve my public speaking skills.

Self-Help Exercise 10.2.
Correcting Negative Anticipatory Thoughts

Evaluate and correct the anxious anticipatory thinking associated with an immediate, weekly, and distant social event using Worksheets 6.3, 6.4, and 6.5. Develop a normalization card for each of these social events. Work on the normalization card throughout the anticipatory period by adding to it and elaborating on various points. In this way you will be correcting your exaggerated anticipatory anxious thinking and reducing your anxiety level. However, it's important not to create a normalization card and then just forget about it. You must continually work on it whenever you feel anxious so that you're actually correcting anticipatory anxious thinking.

≳ Troubleshooting Tips ≲

Even after correcting their exaggerated anxious thinking about a future social event, some people have difficulty coming up with a more helpful way of thinking during the anticipation phase. Asking a close friend or family member what he or she thinks about when nervous about a future event (e.g., job interview, a dinner party with unknown guests) might give you some ideas. Also the alternative, normalized way of thinking must include the fact that you will feel anxious in the event. Trying to convince yourself when you are anticipating a social event that you won't feel anxious won't help because it's just not a realistic expectation.

Dealing with social anxiety in a more constructive manner starts long before you actually engage in a social experience. Working on your anticipatory anxiety by correcting the thinking that fuels anxiety is the best way to prepare for future social situations.

Correcting Negative Postevent Thinking

Looking back on past social experiences can have a major impact on your current level of social anxiety, so it's important to correct thinking about past social experiences that contributes to your anxiety. After you've encountered a social situation, do you tend to think about it for days and days? Do you often go back over events and try to figure out whether it was as awful and embarrassing as you think? Do you try to reassure yourself it wasn't all that bad, but for some reason you can't seem to convince yourself it was okay? Do you end up feeling more convinced that you really "messed up" and are less confident in your ability to handle social situations?

If you answered "yes" to many of these questions, then postevent processing probably plays a critical role in your fear of social situations. It's critical to deal with this phase of the social anxiety cycle (see the diagram on page 199) before you begin exposure to actual social situations. For most people their postevent processing (rumination) will focus on past experiences of "traumatic" embarrassment or humiliation and a more recent experience of anxiety in a social situation.

Step 1: Identify Past and Recent Traumatic Experiences

In the space below, write down one or two past traumatic social experiences that come to your mind whenever you think about your social anxiety. These experiences should involve your worst experience of social anxiety. They may be recent, or they could be events that go back several years, even to your childhood or adolescence. These social events are "the worst thing that has ever happened to you" and usually involve some experience of heightened embarrassment, humiliation, or even feelings of shame.

Most Anxiety-Provoking or Embarrassing Past Social Experience

_____

_____

_____

_____

Now write down the most recent social experiences that you can't seem to get out of your mind. These events may not be as extreme as the "worst social experience," but they do involve anxiety, and you can't stop thinking back and trying to figure out whether the social experience was as bad as you are thinking or why you were so anxious. The important thing is to focus on recent social events that you're still thinking about, that you find yourself ruminating about days or even weeks later.

Recent Social Events

_____

_____

_____

_____

_____

For his most "traumatic" social experience, Martin noted that he had had to give a speech to his ninth-grade class. He said it was the worst day in his life. He was so terrified that he shook uncontrollably and started stuttering. He noticed that some of the students were snickering and the teacher actually stopped him in the middle of the speech and told him to go back to his seat. When he thinks about his problem with social anxiety, he practically relives that terrible experience. For his most recent social events, Martin wrote down several experiences at work, such as having lunch with his coworkers and then worrying that he said something stupid, or having to give a brief to his supervisor and wondering whether he came across as incompetent or poorly prepared.

Once you've identified the social events you find yourself mulling over long after the event ended, it's important to deal with these past memories in a more constructive manner. Let's start with your most recent social experiences. The objective is to discover whether you're exaggerating the negative aspects of the experience and to decatastrophize how you remember the experience so that your thinking is more realistic or balanced. Once again we use the evidence gathering, consequences, and alternative thinking strategies to correct memories of recent social events. There are three things to focus on:

1. Did other people really evaluate you as badly as you remember?

2. Was your anxiety and social performance really as awful as you remember?

3. Are you exaggerating the significance and long-term impact of the experience (i.e., are you catastrophizing)?

Step 2: Gather Evidence for Negative Evaluation

Use the Gathering Evidence form (Worksheet 6.3) to determine whether people in the social situation judged you negatively. Go back over the situation in your mind and write down any comments, nonverbal expressions, or behavior that you interpreted as a negative judgment. Now reevaluate your memory and write down indications that people may have had a positive impression of you at best or a neutral impression at the very least. You could ask a friend present at the situation for his or her observations of how others reacted to you, but you need to be careful that this doesn't become "habit-forming" reassurance seeking. There are three things you need to keep in mind when you do this exercise:

1. *Praise is ephemeral.* What we think about a person changes from moment to moment. So there is no way to earn a "permanent" or guaranteed positive evaluation from other people. It will change from moment to moment depending on individuals' mood state, their circumstances, and other factors.

2. *People are fickle.* Do you really think it's possible for everyone in a social situation to judge you positively? If you say, "No, of course not," then how many people need to hold a positive impression for you to feel good about yourself? Is it really a simple majority, like 51%? Most people with social anxiety have unrealistic beliefs about people's evaluation. Even if 90% of the people at a social event form a reasonably positive impression of you, those one or two people who have a negative impression will outweigh all the positive evaluations. Are you overly focused on one or two people who may have had a negative evaluation? Are there many more people in the social situation who may have had a slightly positive or at least a neutral (i.e., benign) impression of you?

3. *True evaluations are hidden.* Rarely do we tell people what we really think about them. We might smile, nod, and give someone lots of eye contact so they think we're interested in them. But to ourselves we might be thinking "What a bore! I wish she would stop talking," or "How could he be so stupid?" The point is we can never really know what people truly think about us. We don't go around revealing our true feelings about people. If we did, life would be chaotic and extremely stressful. So we keep our thoughts about other people to ourselves. What this means is that in the end you'll *never really know what a person thinks of you.* There is always a big blank about what others truly think of us, and we are all left guessing, filling in the blanks with our preconceived assumptions. The problem in social anxiety is that we always assume that other people think negatively about us.

So with these considerations in mind, what's the evidence that everyone thought badly of you in this social situation? What is the evidence against your negative assumption; the evidence that you are exaggerating how badly others thought of you?

Step 3: Examine the Evidence of Poor Performance

If you have social anxiety, you probably tend to magnify the anxiety of recent social experiences when you think back about them and focus on aspects of your social performance that were ineffective, weak, or even embarrassing. Once again, use Work-sheet 6.3 to examine evidence for and against the view that your anxiety in that situation was intolerable and noticeable to others. Are you overly focused on anxiety symptoms when you remember the situation? Is there any evidence that you managed your anxiety better than you think? Write down indications that other people noticed your anxiety (e.g., any comments or nonverbal stares) as well as evidence that they may not have noticed or even cared whether you were anxious. What can you learn about dealing with your anxiety in similar social situations? What would you do differently the next time?

Step 4: Decatastrophize the Impact

The third question to address is whether you're exaggerating the impact or long-term consequence of the social experience. Use the top half of the Cost–Benefit Analysis form (Worksheet 6.4) to evaluate the impact of the social experience. Let's assume that the social situation really was a "nightmare," that your extreme anxiety showed through, and most people thought you were inappropriate, incompetent, or defective in some way. How has this changed your life? Do your work colleagues, friends, or family now treat you differently? If the "embarrassment" occurred with strangers, how can this change your life? You need to distinguish between the consequences of your social anxiety and the consequences of the event. Right now we're looking at the consequences of the event only. Rarely, except possibly for job interviews or other evaluative situations, does the impression we make on other people have a lasting impact. When we feel embarrassed or anxious in everyday social situations, the actual consequence is usually minimal. The problem is that socially anxious people often treat every social situation, such as a casual conversation, as if it were "life and death." And it's this tendency to exaggerate the importance and significance of social encounters that drives up anxiety. The Cost–Benefit Analysis worksheet is a good way to recalibrate the importance of a social event and see it for what it is: just one of dozens of interpersonal interactions we have in the course of normal daily living.

Step 5: Generate an Alternative

Now that you've evaluated the past social situation and decided that you have been thinking the worst about the situation, it's time to come up with a more realistic account of the social encounter. What is the best, most realistic way to look back on your social experience? Focus on:

■ Developing a new understanding of the social experience.

■ Learning from the social interaction so you can act and think differently when you encounter similar social events in the future.

When generating an alternative perspective, it's important to focus on the facts, what actually happened based on the evidence, rather than on how you feel. You may feel anxious about the situation, but stick to what actually happened when developing your new perspective. What specific details do you remember about what was said to you or how others reacted to you and how you actually behaved in the social situation? Based on these observations, generate an alternative account of the past social experience using Worksheet 10.6, Reevaluating Past Experiences of Social Anxiety.

Once you've done your work on the most recent social events associated with postevent processing, repeat Steps 1–5 for the most traumatic social event you can remember. You might find this a little more challenging because it may have occurred in the distant past and may be associated with a lot of emotion. Nevertheless, it's important to generate a new understanding about these events as well. Once the alternative perspectives have been developed, you can practice replacing the anxious memory of the past events with the alternative, more balanced explanation. This will defuse the anxiety and renew your confidence for facing future social events. It's an effective way to diminish postevent ruminative thinking that can fuel social anxiety.

Self-Help Exercise 10.3.
Correcting Negative Postevent Thinking

Identify a couple of recent social experiences and any past traumatic social events that you continue to fret about. Work through the five-step program just described. Use the results of your cognitive investigation to construct a more realistic, constructive explanation for past social experiences. Each time you start to ruminate about past social experiences, take out your evidence-gathering worksheets as well as Worksheet 10.6 and work on elaborating on the alternative interpretation. Write down why this is the most reasonable way to understand what happened to you. Practice replacing your anxious memories with the more realistic alternative explanation.

Postevent processing played a big role in Marin's social anxiety. On page 221 you can see how Martin filled out Worksheet 10.6. Notice that Martin's alternative explanation did not simply represent more *positive* thinking but the most *realistic* interpretation of the situation. Whenever Martin started worrying about what he had said to his supervisor, he pulled out Worksheet 10.6 and wrote down more evidence for the alternative interpretation and why that is the explanation he should focus on rather than the unrealistic anxious explanation.

Reevaluating Past Experiences of Social Anxiety

Instructions: Based on the evidence gathering and cost–benefit exercises, briefly describe an alternative, more balanced, and constructive interpretation or explanation of the past social experience. First record the past social experience that you still think about and your automatic, most anxious way of remembering it. Then develop an alternative, more constructive explanation and list a few things that you can learn from this experience.

1. Statement of past social experience: _____

_____

2. Initial anxious interpretation of the situation: _____

_____

_____

_____

_____

3. Alternative, constructive interpretation of the situation: _____

_____

_____

_____

_____

4. What I have learned from this situation:

   a. _____

       _____

   b. _____

       _____

   c. _____

       _____

Martin's Reevaluation of a Past Social Anxiety Experience

1. Statement of past social experience: _I keep thinking about last week's meeting with my supervisor (Mr. Smith) and worry about my performance and his opinion of me._

2. Initial anxious interpretation of the situation: _I had a difficult time articulating myself; I know he noticed I was blushing, that my hands were trembling, and that I couldn't express myself clearly. He probably is wondering what's wrong with me, why I was so nervous. He asked several questions, which means I wasn't making sense. I'm so embarrassed; he's probably wondering whether I'm competent enough to do this job._

3. Alternative, constructive interpretation of the situation: _He probably did realize I was nervous but he already knows I'm shy and anxious. He still gives me work to do and frequently asks for my advice. There is plenty of evidence from the nature of his questions that he understood what I was telling him. Since our meeting his behavior toward me has not changed, and he still gives me work and asks my opinion. So obviously he doesn't think I'm incompetent. He can still think I'm competent and even gifted, and possibly even a nice person, but that I have a problem with anxiety. It's likely that he has accepted my anxiety a lot better than I have myself._

4. What I have learned from this situation:

   a. _Expect to be anxious in social situations; accept the anxiety, work with it rather than try to conceal it from others or suppress it._

   b. _Slow down when I talk; I try to rush when I'm anxious because I want to get it over with; this only makes matters worse and harder for people to follow what I am saying._

   c. _Next time ask Mr. Smith in advance the purpose of the meeting; write down a few key points that I can refer to during the meeting._

> ## ⋛ Troubleshooting Tips ⋜
>
> Sometimes the anxiety about a recent social encounter can be so intense that you ruminate about what happened almost constantly throughout the day. If this is happening to you, don't try to suppress or control your anxiety. Let it ebb and flow naturally as you go about your daily tasks. Jot down the things about the social event that you are recalling and then plan to have a special 30- to 60-minute worry session at home in the evening. Take out the things you recorded through the day and work on them using the five-step approach discussed earlier.

Tackling Social Challenges

With the cognitive work just described, you've tackled the pre- and postevent thoughts that contribute to social anxiety. But you have to go out into the social world and gather new evidence that many of the situations in which you've felt anxious are not as threatening as you believed. **Repeated, if not daily, practice entering social situations and interacting with other people is absolutely critical to the rehabilitation of social fear.** To get started on changing your behavior, you will probably find it useful to review Chapter 7.

Behavioral change that can reduce your social fears and transform your interactions with others involves four tasks.

In cognitive therapy we use evidence gathering, cost–benefit analysis, and generating an alternative perspective to reduce negative postevent processing. But they're not enough on their own: you also need to expose yourself to new social situations and use the evidence from them to challenge anxious thinking and reinforce the alternative.

Step 1: Construct a Social Action Plan

Taking concrete steps to overcome your social anxiety involves courageously exposing yourself to the source of your anxiety—the fear you experience when around people. We can't emphasize enough that applying the behavioral strategies in Chapter 7 to your feared social situations is a **necessary component** of cognitive therapy for social anxiety.

Self-Help Exercise 10.4.
Constructing and Implementing a Social Action Plan

If you included social situations on the Exposure Hierarchy form in Chapter 7 (Worksheet 7.3), you should review this form as the first step in constructing your social anxiety profile. (If you did not complete Worksheet 7.3, you should do that now, before continuing.) Select a situation that is three or four items from the bottom—one that causes you mild to moderate anxiety and occurs at least two or three times a week. Then construct an exposure plan using the five steps for constructing an effective exposure plan discussed in Chapter 7 (pages 132–139). Worksheet 10.7 presents a form you can use to record your social anxiety exposure plan.

Martin selected "join coworkers for casual conversation at coffee break" as his first exposure task. Using Worksheet 10.7, Martin wrote down specific details of the exposure task: "Attend the 10:30 A.M. coffee break for 15 minutes at least three days a week, sit around the table with coworkers, and mainly listen. Think of one comment you can make on the main topic of conversation." He noted that the typical anxious thoughts he had to watch out for were "Everyone is looking at me," "They will notice I'm blushing," and "They probably think I'm such a loser because I'm so quiet." For his correct alternative thinking, Martin wrote, "These people already know me well, so there is nothing I'm going to say or not say during a coffee break that will significantly change their opinion of me," "It's okay to be quiet and a person of few words—there are others like me in the office," and "Just be myself—a quiet and somewhat nervous guy—because everyone already knows this about me and they seem to accept me; I really don't have anything to lose at this point." In terms of safety-seeking behaviors, Martin reminded himself that he needs to work on eye contact and to reduce his tendency to look down at the floor. He also decided to leave his water bottle back at his office cubicle and instead join the others and have a cup of coffee. For useful coping strategies he would concentrate on what other people were saying, try to notice whether anyone else appeared self-conscious, take a couple of relaxing breaths before he spoke, and wear more comfortable clothing because he knew he would feel hot from anxiety.

After writing out his detailed exposure plan, Martin began attending at least three coffee breaks over the next week. He recorded each exposure on the Exposure Practice form (Worksheet 7.4) and noticed that his anxiety decreased greatly over time. By the end of 3 weeks, Martin felt minimal anxi-

Social Anxiety Exposure

Instructions: Complete this worksheet by following the steps in developing an exposure plan described in Chapter 7.

Description of social exposure plan: _____

_____

_____

_____

Typical anxious thinking to modify: _____

_____

_____

_____

Alternative corrected thinking to adopt: _____

_____

_____

_____

Maladaptive safety & control behaviors to eliminate: _____

_____

_____

_____

Useful coping strategies to implement: _____

_____

_____

_____

ety during coffee breaks and couldn't believe this had been such a difficult social situation for him just a few weeks earlier.

≳ Troubleshooting Tips ≲

The hardest part of exposure is getting started. Sometimes people start with social situations that are too easy, and so they end up making little progress because they are doing things they would probably do anyway. At the other extreme are people who start with tasks too challenging and so become quickly overwhelmed with anxiety and discouragement, and then they give up. To ensure that you are starting off exposure with the best chance of success, you could consult with your therapist or your spouse, a close friend, or a family member who knows about your social anxiety to get his or her opinion on a good realistic first exposure assignment. It is important that the assignment be challenging but not overwhelming. You don't want to defeat yourself before you get started.

Facing your social fears to practice correcting the faulty thoughts and behaviors that maintain social anxiety begins with writing out specific exposure assignments that you can follow regularly over the coming weeks.

Step 2: Correct Unrealistic Expectations

Negative thinking and unrealistic expectations can defeat your best efforts at exposure. Read over the following list and check any of the expectations that you may hold about doing exposure. You can add to the list other expectations that may be unique to you but might undermine the success of your exposure tasks.

☐ After completing all of these workbook exercises, I should be so well prepared that I won't feel anxious in the exposure situation.

☐ I should be able to suppress the anxiety and conceal my nervousness from others.

☐ I'm certain people will notice that I'm nervous or awkward and will think I'm incompetent, inept, or defective in some way.

☐ I need to make a good impression on other people so they'll think I'm interesting, intelligent, or witty.

☐ I should be much more assertive and appear confident around people.

☐ It's my responsibility to keep the conversation going.

☐ My conversation or communication with others needs to be clear, concise, and effective.

☐ I need to feel I'm in control at all times.

☐ For an exposure assignment to be successful, I need to be positive and feel good about myself.

☐ I need to feel I've been effective with other people or that the exercise was highly successful to benefit from a social exposure assignment.

☐ I need to experience some signs of approval or acceptance from other people to benefit from a social exposure task.

☐ I must feel that I'm wanted and accepted by others present in the social situation.

So what is the most helpful, alternative attitude to have about exposure? It's important to realize you'll feel anxious during exposure to the social situation, you probably won't come across to others as well as you would like, and some people probably will detect that you're feeling a little uncomfortable or even nervous. Also, you probably will feel awkward, different from others, and not particularly well accepted in the social situation. No doubt you'll feel self-conscious and come away from the social interaction aware of weaknesses in your social performance. But the important thing to remember about exposure is that you're facing your social fears and you'll conquer them with PRACTICE, PRACTICE, PRACTICE. It's critical to be realistic with yourself about what to expect when doing exposure. If your expectations are unrealistic, you will quickly be disappointed with your exposure attempts and give up on the therapy.

> Unrealistic expectations can easily undermine your exposure efforts. Your goals for each exposure should be practical and realistic: provide an opportunity to face your fear of a specific social situation, correct faulty beliefs that maintain your social anxiety, and learn to improve your interpersonal skills.

Before each exposure task, do a mental check of your expectations. You might be surprised at how easily these unrealistic expectations and wishes creep back into your mind. If you find yourself hoping that the exposure will unfold in an unrealistic fashion, correct it by doing a reality check, reminding yourself of the alternative perspective (that you will be anxious, etc.), which is more practical and is firmly anchored in reality.

Step 3: Implement Cognitive Strategies

There are several cognitive strategies you can use during exposure to a feared social situation that will help with your anxiety level:

Maintain an External Focus

To break the habit of being overly attentive to your internal emotional state and sensations, deliberately and consciously take note of other people. Pay attention to what people are saying. You might have to repeat to yourself what they are saying to make sure you're tracking what is being said.

Look for Positive Social Cues

To counter your sensitivity to signs of threat or disapproval, intentionally seek out positive cues from others. Focus on the person who looks interested, who has a positive facial expression, and is paying attention to your conversation. Both of us are university professors and have given hundreds of lectures to students, professionals, and the general public. As a speaker you learn quickly to focus on the one or two students who look interested in your lecture and to pay as little attention as possible to the students who are sleeping, texting, or look utterly bored with your talk. This is the number-one survival tip of the professional public speaker!

Minimize Thinking Errors

Many of the thinking errors discussed in Chapter 3 dominate when we expose ourselves to social fear situations. Mind-reading (assuming we know what other people are thinking), jumping to conclusions, tunnel vision, and all-or-nothing thinking are common mistakes. Learning to identify these errors and reminding yourself that the way you see the situation is probably biased and overly negative is an important therapeutic strategy to practice. The most important fact to keep in mind is **that none of us can be sure what other people think of us or can control what other people think of us.** We all have to accept there is much that is unknown and beyond our control in social situations. Trying to guess at what people are really thinking about us is fertile ground for thinking errors to creep into our conclusions.

Correct Exaggerated Threat Appraisals

In social situations the anxious person will tend to think that the probability and severity of other people's rejection, disapproval, or negative judgment is much greater than it really is. Recognizing your tendency to exaggerate the negative and learning to recalibrate your evaluations so they are closer to reality will be a significant factor in reducing your anxiety level.

One of the best ways to overcome a fear of other people is learning to counter the biased thinking about the negative evaluation and disapproval of others that fuels social anxiety.

Self-Help Exercise 10.5.
Practicing in Less Anxiety-Provoking Situations

Implementing cognitive strategies to correct biased thinking can be very difficult when one is intensely anxious. One way to overcome this problem is to practice these skills in non-anxiety-provoking or mildly uncomfortable situations. You can practice directing your attention to other people, processing the positive cues in your social environment, catching cognitive errors, and correcting biased threat-related evaluations in these less intimidating situations. With dozens of practice trials these cognitive skills will become more and more automatic so you will begin using them even when you're in high-anxiety situations.

⋛ Troubleshooting Tips ⋚

If you have difficulty correcting your anxious thinking in social situations, try breaking down the problem. Identify one specific anxious thought (e.g., "I am drawing attention to myself") and work on correcting it rather than every anxious thought you are having in the situation. Next decide on which cognitive strategy you will use to counter this anxious thought and then practice using the strategy against the anxious thought. Once you've made progress on this thought, move on to another anxious thought and try using another cognitive strategy.

Step 4: Use Behavioral Strategies

Overcoming anxiety in social situations will not occur without significant changes in behavior. You must repeatedly expose yourself to feared social situations, employing various new behavioral strategies that will help reduce your anxiety level. The following list presents some behavioral strategies that are useful for reducing social anxiety, bolstering self-confidence, and improving social performance.

- ■ Practice using role plays and behavioral rehearsal before actual exposure.
- ■ Videotape role plays and then evaluate your performance.
- ■ Identify safety behaviors and gradually eliminate them.
- ■ Refine verbal communication skills.

■ Modify problematic nonverbal behaviors.

■ Practice assertiveness skills.

■ Learn to manage confrontation, anger, and criticism from others.

Role Playing

Cognitive therapists do a lot of role playing when treating social anxiety. Therapist and client role-play various social situations the client experiences in her everyday circumstances. New ways of interacting can be practiced, and the therapist can run through various worst-case scenarios a person is concerned might happen, such as dealing with an angry or critical response from people or handling potential embarrassment. Also, role plays are a great way to elicit automatic anxious thoughts that can be corrected on the spot. If you are not in therapy, you can still use role plays to prepare yourself for anxiety-provoking social situations. You could do role plays with your spouse, a family member, or a close friend. In fact it will be more effective if you have two or three people to do role plays with you. This will introduce some variation and novelty into the practice sessions. Martin, for example, wanted to ask a woman colleague out for a date but was petrified even thinking about it. He worked with his therapist on how to initiate a conversation with her. They spent a considerable amount of time repeatedly role-playing how to strike up a casual conversation, working on Martin's communication skills and strategies for interacting with others even when feeling intensely anxious.

Videotape Self-Evaluation

Videotape can make your role plays even more effective in two ways: First, videotaping gives you immediate feedback about your performance so you can pick out specific behaviors you may want to work on, such as making more eye contact, increasing your speech volume, or expressing attentive nonverbal behaviors when people are speaking to you (nodding in agreement, etc.). Second, videotaping can help you correct biased negative evaluations about your social performance and how you think you appear to others. Professor David M. Clark (no relation), an expert in social anxiety at the Institute of Psychiatry in London, England, has individuals with social anxiety discuss how they think they appear to others when they watch their videotaped role play.[42] The therapist and client then evaluate this observation of "how I think I appear to others" and correct overly negative or pessimistic interpretations.

Martin would look at his videotaped performance of casual conversation and think, "I look like a total nerd; people must be thinking I'm mentally unstable." Of course, this type of thinking was not only biased and inaccurate but also made Martin feel substantially more anxious when speaking with others. Martin and his therapist were able to correct this biased interpretation through use of videotape role plays. If you are not in therapy, you can use videotape to correct biased thinking by first observing the videotaped role play alone and writing down how you think you appear to the other person. Then have a friend or family member watch the tape and write her observation of how you come across to other people. Now compare your observations. Are you being overly negative about your performance and how you think you appear to others? If so, it's important to correct this interpretation before you expose yourself to the social situation.

Eliminating Safety Behavior

Looking down, mumbling, holding a rigid body posture, having a drink, taking deep breaths, continually consulting your notes, clearing your throat repeatedly, wearing dark sunglasses, and displaying other signs of inhibition may give you the illusion of managing your anxiety in the short term, but often these behaviors make social interactions more inhibited and awkward, actually drawing more attention to you. Martin, for example, would take "relaxing" breaths when he became intensely anxious, but these came across as deep sighs that were annoying to other people trying to talk to him. If it's hard for you to identify your safety behaviors, have a friend observe you in social situations and note anything you might be doing quite automatically that interrupts the flow of your social interaction. Of course if you're in therapy, your cognitive therapist will work with you on reducing your safety behavior.

Behavioral Rehearsal

The remaining behavioral strategies in the preceding list all involve learning to refine specific social skills. Improving your verbal communication, being more assertive, and dealing better with anger, conflict, or criticism from others all can ease social anxiety. Once again role plays and videotaping are indispensable for identifying weaknesses in your social performance and practicing new social skills. Don't try to change too many behaviors at once. Select one or two specific behaviors such as improving eye contact, speaking more loudly, or learning to interrupt others in a polite manner so you are not left out of conversations. Work on these behaviors and give yourself opportunities to practice them in actual social situations before moving on to another behavioral weakness you want to improve. Also try out these new behaviors in repeated role plays and in non-anxiety-provoking social situations so they become much more automatic even when you feel intense anxiety. Above all, *be kind to yourself.* Don't expect too much too quickly. Behavioral change takes a lot of time and practice. Many habits you may be trying to break have been with you for a lifetime. Don't expect to break a lifelong habit in a couple of weeks. Be realistic with yourself and give yourself credit when you've made changes and faced your daunting social fears.[28]

Self-Help Exercise 10.6. Using Role Plays and Social Skills Practice

Select a moderately anxiety-provoking social situation from your social fear hierarchy. Ask a friend or your spouse to engage in role plays of this situation with you (doing a job interview, speaking up at a meeting, etc). Make sure you do the role play several times a week. Ask your role-play partner for feedback on any safety behaviors that may be evident during your role play. Correct any exaggerated negative thoughts you may have about your role-play performance and practice one or two specific social skills. Develop a normalization card for dealing with this social situation. After several role-play practices, engage in the actual social activity and record the outcome on your Monitoring Your Social Anxiety form (Worksheet 10.5).

≳ Troubleshooting Tips ≲

Role playing is another name for acting, and some people find it very difficult to act, that is, to pretend to be someone else. Instead of acting out their role, they comment on the role (i.e., they talk about what they should say rather than pretending to actually say it). If this is happening to you, try writing out a script first—a set of lines to say just like an actor's script. Now try acting out the lines by saying them as if you were actually in the feared social situation. Eventually you should work up to being more spontaneous and not reading lines when you practice role-playing the social situation.

The most effective way to overcome social anxiety is to engage in role play prior to a social interaction and then repeatedly expose yourself to the actual social situation. In the end your exposure experiences to real-life anxiety-provoking social situations will radically alter your anxiety and bolster your self-confidence around other people.

CHAPTER SUMMARY

■ Social anxiety is characterized by (1) fear of negative evaluation by others, (2) heightened self-focus on symptoms of anxiety and social performance, and (3) extensive avoidance of social situations.

■ It is quite normal to feel some anxiety or discomfort in unfamiliar social situations or when performing in public, such as making a speech. However, when the anxiety is so intense and persistent that it causes avoidance of common, everyday social experiences and interferes in one's quality of life, it has become a psychological problem that can be treated with the cognitive therapy approach.

■ Social anxiety builds during anticipation, actual exposure, and postevent remembrance of social experiences because of biased thinking that (1) exaggerates the probability and severity of negative evaluation by others, (2) is overly self-focused on the symptoms of anxiety and their concealment, (3) relies on safety behaviors to suppress anxious feelings, and (4) overestimates the sense of embarrassment, shame, and humiliation related to one's performance in social situations.

■ Reducing your social anxiety starts with developing your social anxiety profile: constructing a hierarchy of social situations, monitoring your anxious thoughts during anticipation and actual exposure to social experiences, determining the automatic coping responses produced when you feel anxious, and discovering what social experiences you tend to recall and how they are interpreted when you think back on past social events.

■ Learning to correct biased thinking and expectations during the anticipation of social encounters is one of the first problems dealt with in cognitive therapy for social anxiety. It is important to develop realistic and adaptive expectations that will prepare you for social situations.

■ Correcting biased memories and false interpretations about past "traumatic" and more recent social experiences is critical to building self-confidence and reducing social anxiety about similar events in the future. Identification, evidence gathering, decatastrophizing, and generating alternative perspectives are cognitive strategies used to gain a more realistic view of your past social experiences.

■ Reducing anxiety and boosting self-confidence in actual social situations involves constructing a social action plan, correcting unrealistic expectations, implementing adaptive cognitive strategies, and adopting various behavioral interventions like preparatory role playing, videotaped behavioral rehearsal, and elimination of safety behaviors.

■ Overcoming social anxiety will take time, lots of practice implementing the strategies discussed in this chapter, and a gradual approach as you work toward conquering some of your greatest social fears. Throughout this process, be kind to yourself; give yourself credit when you make progress, and try to learn from your mistakes. Fear of people can be an incapacitating condition, but over the years thousands of people have gained a new lease on life from defeating their social anxiety with the research-based cognitive and behavioral strategies presented in this chapter.

11

Overcoming Worry

This chapter is especially relevant for you if:

- Your anxiety occurs primarily in the form of worry and remains a problem even though you've worked through the Anxiety Work Plan you created in Chapter 8.

- You've been a chronic worrier and you tend to worry about many different things in your life.

- You meet most of the diagnostic criteria for generalized anxiety disorder.

- You are having difficulty falling asleep because of worry (i.e., a racing mind).

Sylvia is a "worry wart," or at least that's the reputation she has with her friends, family, and coworkers. A married 57-year-old mother of two adult sons, a senior partner in an accounting firm, a committed community activist, and a prospective grandmother expecting her first grandchild, even Sylvia describes herself as an anxious person with a penchant for expecting the worst. Ever since high school she has worried about the possibility of impending doom. Now she worries about anything and everything—her own health and her husband's, the recent decline in her financial investments and the looming prospect of retirement, her work performance, her daughter-in-law's pregnancy, her younger son's search for a new job, their plans to remodel a bathroom, even getting the housework done. She has tried a number of interventions over the years, from antidepressants and tranquilizers to repeated sessions with various mental health professionals, to yoga, meditation, nutrition programs, fairly strenuous aerobic exercise, and the like, but nothing seems to work. As the years advance her worry only seems to get worse, and now Sylvia feels trapped, with worry robbing her of what she thought would be "the best years of my life."

Sylvia suffers from pathological worry that is the central characteristic of a condition called *generalized anxiety disorder* (GAD). Worry is a common experience in most people's lives, but the excessive worry associated with GAD is much more severe, persistent, and uncontrollable than "normal worry." GAD worry can last for hours, occurs almost daily, and involves multiple concerns. It typically takes a chronic course, lasting several months but more often several years or even decades. People with this type of excessive worry are generally anxious so they often feel more tired, frustrated, tense, distracted, restless, and sleep deprived. Together with their excessive worry, this state of generalized anxiety can disrupt one's normal daily functioning.

In the last two decades psychologists and psychiatrists have learned a great deal about worry. With these insights and a modified form of cognitive therapy based on them, we can offer new hope for those caught in the grip of excessive and unproductive worry. In this chapter we pinpoint factors that contribute to the *persistence of worry* and describe cognitive and behavioral strategies that can improve your control over the worry process. You can expect to gain a better understanding of worry and a more effective approach to worry control if you do the work in this chapter in addition to what you did in Chapters 1–8.

Understanding Generalized Anxiety

GAD is very common, affecting more than 700,000 adult Americans (3.1%) in a given year,[1] tends to be chronic, and even seems like a personality characteristic to many sufferers, who report always having been anxious and worried. Perhaps this accounts for why it can be a difficult anxiety problem to treat. Medication and standard psychological treatment have shown an effectiveness rate of only about 50%,[43] although recovery rates have been quite variable across studies and we still have limited information on the long-term effectiveness of treatment. Antianxiety medications can be effective in reducing generalized anxiety in the short term, but they tend to lose their effectiveness after several weeks and can be difficult to discontinue when a person develops physical and/or psychological dependence.[44] Antidepressant medication can also be effective and is probably the pharmacological treatment of choice for GAD, but relapse rates approach 50% after 6 months of stopping the medication.[44] However, progress is being made, and there is encouraging evidence that the newer forms of cognitive therapy that focus on the specific features of GAD discussed in this chapter may improve treatment outcome[45] and help people get off their antianxiety medication.[46]

Why Do We Worry?

To get a handle on chronic worrying, we have to start with an understanding of what we mean by worry. For the purposes of this book, *worry* is:

a persistent, repetitive, and uncontrollable chain of thinking that mainly focuses on the uncertainty of some future negative or threatening outcome in which the person rehearses various problem-solving solutions but fails to reduce the heightened sense of uncertainty about the possible threat.

We can worry about a wide variety of things, from the most inconsequential daily task (such as getting to a hair appointment on time) to very significant personal tragedies (having a terminal illness) to major world affairs (failing to deal with climate change). No two people have exactly the same worry concerns, but as evidenced by Sylvia, many of us worry about serious matters like our health, the potential for injury to or death of a loved one, our finances, work, and the state of the world. We also worry about all kinds of trivial things, like the logistics of daily schedules and routine tasks. Using Worksheet 11.1, write down any present and recurring worry concerns you have in various life domains.

As with every other type of anxiety, a certain amount of worry is normal. So how does worry become persistent and uncontrollable for some people? Why are some people better able to control their worries than others, such as those with GAD, who seem paralyzed by the worry process? The following are features of excessive worry that account for its persistence and uncontrollability.

- **Catastrophizing:** Exclusive focus on the possibility of a highly negative, disturbing, or threatening future outcome.

- **Heightened anxiety:** Worry process associated with personal sense of anxiousness or nervousness that can involve physical symptoms like muscle tension, feeling on edge, restlessness, and so forth.

- **Intolerance of uncertainty:** Difficulty accepting the uncertainty of future events and so striving to gain assurance that the imagined dreaded catastrophe won't happen.

- **Difficulty accepting risk:** Attempts to eliminate or at least minimize any possibility of future danger, disappointment, or failure.

- **Futile problem solving:** Repeated efforts to prepare an effective response to an imagined catastrophe but feeling dissatisfied with each potential solution generated.

- **Striving for perfection:** Attempts to find a perfect solution for the imagined negative event that will bring relief and a sense of personal safety or security.

- **Failed worry control:** Repeated efforts to stop worry that are ineffective and actually strengthen the worry process.

- **Dysfunctional worry-related beliefs:** Maladaptive beliefs about the positive and

Worry Across the Life Domains

Instructions: Write down any current worries you have within any of the following important life domains. If you don't have any worries in a domain, leave it blank.

1. Health (self): _____

   _____

2. Health (family, friends): _____

   _____

3. Safety concerns (self, children, family): _____

   _____

4. Work or school: _____

   _____

5. Finances: _____

   _____

6. Intimate relationships: _____

   _____

7. Other relationships (family, friendships, work colleagues): _____

   _____

8. Minor matters (e.g., making appointments, completing daily chores): _____

   _____

9. Community, world affairs (e.g., global warming, terrorist attacks): _____

   _____

10. Spiritual matters: _____

   _____

negative effects of worry and its controllability may be an important cause of worry.

■ **Worry about worry:** The process of worrying about not being able to control worry can intensify the whole process.

Let's say you work for a company that is experiencing economic difficulties and has already laid off many employees. It would be perfectly natural and realistic to wonder, "Am I next? Will I lose my job as well?" But how you think about this concern will determine whether you shift from normal worry to a persistent and uncontrollable state of worry that causes significant distress and interference in your life.

Based on the preceding list of contributing factors, we can outline a way of thinking about the possibility of unemployment that would make it a persistent and uncontrollable concern. You could begin by catastrophizing, thinking only about the 20% of employees who lost their job rather than the 80% still working for the company. You could refuse to accept that the future is uncertain and unknowable, that both good and bad events happen without our ability to forecast their occurrence. You could

> Cognitive therapy targets the core features of the worry process that contribute to its escalation so that you can learn different strategies for gaining better control.

continually remind yourself that you hate risks, and so you could endlessly try to think about how you'll deal with unemployment. Of course, anything you come up with seems frightening and unsatisfactory, so you keep going around in circles. You try hard not to worry, but it doesn't stop, and you end up feeling even more anxious and discouraged. You're thinking that you should be worried about losing your job, that it's better to be prepared for the worst than to be blindsided by it, but the worry is relentless, and now you're afraid that it's having a negative impact on your health and work performance. You worry about being so worried, that your worry could lead to the very thing you fear—loss of your job. And so you remain stuck in a pathological process of worry.

Do We Worry Because Sometimes It's Productive?

Psychologists agree that most worry is useless at best and counterproductive at worst, because we can waste so much time and endure so much misery dealing with the *what ifs* that we don't enjoy any aspect of the present moment—and most of the time the object of our worry doesn't materialize anyway. Yet our history is filled with cautionary tales about what happens when one doesn't "worry" about the future and thus ends up unprepared for predictable challenges. So where is the line between constructive and unconstructive worry? Table 11.1 presents a number of key differences between unproductive and productive worry.

Let's examine Sylvia's worry about her bathroom remodeling. When she thinks

TABLE 11.1. **Characteristics of Unproductive and Productive Worry**

Unproductive worry	Productive worry
• Focus on distant, imagined "what if" scenarios	• Focus on more immediate, realistic problems
• Focus on imagined problems that we have little control or ability to influence	• Focus on impending problems over which we have some control or influence
• Tendency to focus on how upset we would feel if the worry concern actually happened	• Greater focus on problem-solving the worry concern
• Failure to accept any solution for the worry concern because it cannot guarantee success	• Can try out and evaluate less than perfect solutions to the worry concern
• Relentless pursuit of a sense of safety and certainty about the imagined outcome	• Willingness to tolerate reasonable risk and uncertainty
• A very narrow and exaggerated focus on the imagined threat or worst-case scenario (i.e., catastrophizing)	• A broader, more balanced focus on all aspects of the worry concern; the ability to recognize the positive, negative, and benign aspects of the situation
• A feeling of helplessness to cope with the worry situation	• A greater degree of self-confidence in one's ability to cope with worry situation
• High levels of anxiety or distress	• Low anxiety or distress

Note. Based on *Cognitive Therapy of Anxiety Disorders* by David A. Clark and Aaron T. Beck (Table 10.6, p. 427). Copyright 2010 by The Guilford Press.[5]

about the bathroom renovations, which she does every day, Sylvia becomes completely stuck on highly negative scenarios like "What if the contractors we hired are incompetent and do a poor job?" and "What if they don't listen to what we want and we end up with renovations we hate?" and "What if they get started and then leave for weeks on end to do other jobs?" and "What if we go way over our budget?" She tries to think about various ways to deal with the contractors that will guarantee they will keep to their schedule, do the job to her satisfaction, and not run over on costs. But nothing seems to help, and she ends up with a sick feeling in her stomach that the whole project will be a disaster. She tries to stop worrying by reminding herself that it's just a bathroom renovation and everything will be fine, but she can't convince herself. She begins to worry that her uncontrolled worry about even the most mundane matters is taking a toll on her health and that she will end up having a "nervous breakdown" or a heart attack from all the stress.

If Sylvia engaged in "productive worry" about the bathroom renovation, her thinking process would look much different. She would go through a checklist to remind herself what she has done to hire the most competent contractor (e.g., checked references, obtained a detailed work estimate, signed a contract). She would talk with friends who had done similar renovations and would work on learning to live with the risk and uncertainty of hiring contractors. She could remind herself that there are lots of things in her house she would like to change but has been able to live with, so if she is not 100% satisfied with the bathroom renovation, she can live with that as well. She would also focus on the fact that any improvements will be better than the existing bathroom, which she has lived with for years. If the contractors renege on the contract, she has legal avenues for dealing with that problem. Finally, she will reframe the problem and remind herself that a new bathroom has little impact on her life satisfaction and meaning. Even if she feels a little apprehensive about launching into a bathroom renovation at this time, she'll normalize these feelings and accept them, realizing that most people feel uneasy when they spend a significant amount of money.

> Cognitive therapy can teach you how to turn the excessive, unproductive worry that is the central problem in generalized anxiety into a more productive, realistic way to think about the possibility of future problems or difficulties.

Worksheet 11.2 contains 10 statements about worry that you can use to determine whether you suffer from unproductive worry. If a majority of the statements apply to you, it's likely that your worry is excessive and unproductive and you'll want to put the extra time into working through this chapter.

The Worried Mind

It's obvious to everyone that worry is all about how we think, so it should be no surprise that cognitive therapy can help with this problem. To benefit from this approach, though, you need to understand how the worried mind operates. A diagram that illustrates the cognitive model of worry is on page 241.

There are three phases to worry: (1) the occurrence of distressing intrusive thoughts, (2) activation of negative beliefs, and (3) the actual worry process itself. In cognitive therapy we focus on negative beliefs that underlie worry and critical features of the worry process (worry about worry, failed problem solving, mental control efforts, and search for relief).

Distressing Intrusive Thoughts Phase

We all experience troubling thoughts or images that suddenly pop into our mind, become the focus of our attention, and interrupt whatever task we're doing. The thoughts, images, or memories literally *intrude into conscious awareness*. These mental intruders may be about irrelevant, even silly things, and we easily ignore them, or we might say to ourselves "That's weird—why did I just think about that?" (I just had

"Worry Wart" Checklist

Instructions: Review the main worry concerns you recorded on Worksheet 11.1. Read through the following items and consider *how you worry* when you think about these concerns. Circle "yes" if the statement characterizes how you *tend to worry* about the things you listed in Worksheet 11.1 or "no" if the statement does not apply. If you circled "yes" to a majority of the items, you probably suffer from unproductive worry.

1. When I worry, I get stuck on the most negative possibility (*what if*s) of the situation.	Yes	No
2. When I worry, I tend to think about how upset I will feel if this situation actually happens.	Yes	No
3. When I worry, I keep trying to figure out what I can do to prevent the worst-case scenario.	Yes	No
4. When I worry, I keep trying to convince myself the worst-case scenario won't happen, but I can never feel assured or convinced that everything will be all right.	Yes	No
5. When I worry, I come up with various responses or solutions to the problem, but I end up rejecting them all because they don't seem adequate to deal with the situation.	Yes	No
6. When I worry, "not knowing" about the future bothers me most.	Yes	No
7. During worry episodes I feel so helpless and ill prepared to deal with life's difficulties.	Yes	No
8. Despite my best efforts, I end up feeling frustrated and discouraged with my inability to stop worrying.	Yes	No
9. When I worry, I keep trying to work out what is the most likely outcome of this situation, but I am always left feeling uncertain.	Yes	No
10. I often think about how miserable my life will be if I don't get a handle on this worry.	Yes	No

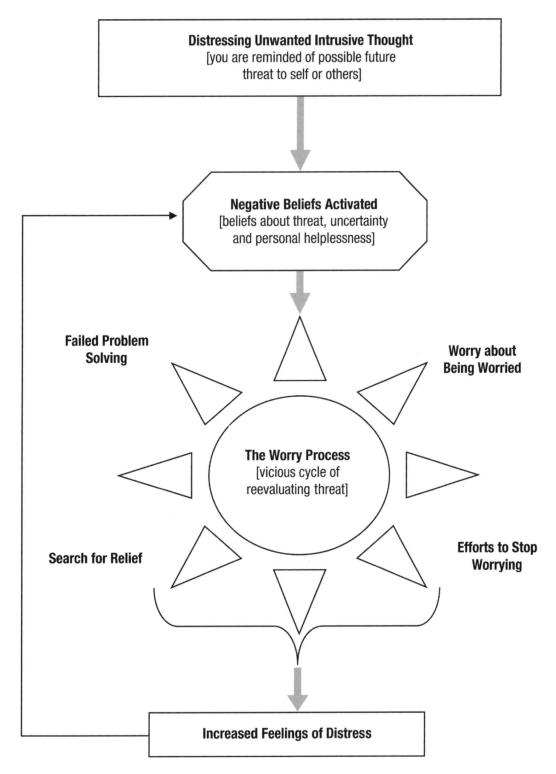

The cognitive model of worry.

a thought about melting snow—strange, even stupid, certainly irrelevant, and easily ignored so I can get back to writing!)

However, not all intrusive thoughts are stupid, random thoughts. Some of these intrusions are *what if* thoughts about the future, and often they involve the possibility of some future threat, danger, or negative outcome. The following are some examples of a distressing, future-based intrusive thought or image that could start a worry episode:

- Thinking of going into next week's meeting without your report ready.
- Remembering a friend telling you she saw your husband with another woman at a restaurant.
- Being reminded of the bank foreclosing on your mortgage.
- Imagining that your child is seriously injured at daycare.
- Remembering the doctor telling you of a positive test for breast cancer.
- Thinking of meeting with an important client and saying something really stupid or embarrassing.
- Thinking that people are looking at you.
- Imagining the house is a disaster and the neighbors arrive unexpectedly for a visit.
- Thinking about your investment losses.

The average person has dozens, maybe even hundreds, of intrusive thoughts in a typical day, involving everything from mundane, trivial issues to really serious, important, and even life-threatening matters. Most of the time we ignore or easily dismiss our intrusive thoughts, but occasionally a thought will grab our attention and we can't let go of it. These attention-grabbing intrusive thoughts and images can start the worry process.

Worry-related intrusive thoughts have three characteristics:

1. *High personal relevance.* They typically deal with matters that are really important to us; they are highly relevant to our personal goals, values, and concerns. For example, only a highly devout religious person would pay attention to an intrusive thought about being earnest and sincere in his praying.

2. *Exaggerated threat.* The intrusive thought involves some negative outcome that is quite extreme. We don't worry over intrusive thoughts that represent mildly distressing or inconvenient outcomes. Rather it is the thought of some impending catastrophe to self or loved ones that grabs our attention.

3. *Cued thoughts.* Often worry-related intrusions are triggered by circumstances or information encountered during our daily activities. A television commercial, a remark at the office, something noticed on the way home from work … we process millions of cues that could trigger an intrusive thought. Sylvia would hear a baby cry, think about her daughter-in-law's pregnancy, and then start worrying about the health of the unborn child.

What types of intrusive thoughts have you experienced that may have started you worrying about some important issue in your life? Complete Worksheet 11.3 to identify distressing intrusive thoughts or images you may experience that cause you to worry. Understanding why you suffer from persistent and uncontrollable worry begins with determining the source of your worry concerns.

> The worry process usually begins with an unwanted distressing intrusive thought that suddenly pops into your mind and reflects a threat to a valued goal or personal striving—an issue of high personal significance.

Activation of Negative Beliefs Phase

At the heart of the worried mind lies a set of negative beliefs that is the engine of the worry process. Even though you may barely be aware of their existence, these beliefs are very real, and they determine whether worry escalates into an uncontrollable, dominating vicious cycle. As explained in Chapter 3, anxious beliefs are often learned during childhood or adolescence and then reinforced by life experiences throughout adulthood. Table 11.2 presents the four types of beliefs that are responsible for uncontrollable worry. Read through this table and circle any beliefs that seem particularly relevant to your worry. In the space provided at the bottom, add any beliefs you have that are probably relevant to your worry concerns. We'll discuss how to identify your worry-related beliefs more in the next section.

Sylvia's problem with worry was based on a number of problematic beliefs. When she worried about retirement, she was convinced they wouldn't have enough money to make ends meet even though she and her husband had good retirement savings. She could only think about having to sell the house and move into a tiny apartment.

> Uncontrollable worry is activated by certain negative beliefs about the worry process that can be revealed and corrected in cognitive therapy.

At her age, she could not figure out any solution other than working well into her 70s. She repeatedly sought financial advice and talked to her husband endlessly about how they could afford retirement, but in the absence of a "crystal ball" that would show her happy and secure, nothing eased her worry about the future. Sylvia believed that her worry about retirement meant that she was taking it seriously and that it prevented

Personal Concerns and Worry–Related Intrusive Thoughts

Instructions: Write down four or five concerns that you would consider highly important personal goals, values, or personal strivings. Examples might be attaining a highly successful or productive career, having a number of close and caring friends, sharing your life with a strong and loving intimate partner, keeping in good physical health and well-being, or maintaining a strong spiritual faith. In the second column, write down some upsetting intrusive thoughts related to that personal striving that you have experienced or could experience. These thoughts would grab your attention because they threaten the personal goal or striving.

Personal Striving, Goal, Value	Examples of Threatening Intrusive Thoughts
1.	
2.	
3.	
4.	
5.	

TABLE 11.2. **Negative Beliefs That Fuel Worry**

Types of worrying beliefs	Examples
1. *Exaggerated threat* (beliefs that worst-case scenarios are likely to happen and so you need to be prepared for them)	• "I won't have enough time to properly prepare this presentation; I could really mess up!" • "The roads are icy; John could have a serious car accident!" • "I've lost a lot of money in the stock market; what if I never rebuild my investments before I retire?" • "What if the test for cancer turns out to be positive?" • "Now that I'm unemployed, what if I never find another decent job?"
2. *Personal helplessness* (beliefs about one's inability to cope effectively with future negative outcomes)	• "I couldn't handle being alone the rest of my life." • "I can't stand making mistakes or not succeeding at everything I do." • "There is nothing I can do to obtain love and acceptance." • "I am struck with my utter helplessness to ensure good health." • "I have no control over what happens to my loved ones."
3. *Intolerance of uncertainty* (beliefs that the uncertainty or ambiguity of future negative events should be minimized as much as possible)	• "I can't stand not knowing how it will turn out." • "It's important to be prepared for the worst even if it is unlikely to happen." • "If I can only be reassured that everything will be fine, then it probably will be fine." • "The more uncertain a future outcome, the more likely it will turn out negatively."
4. *Beliefs about the worry process* (beliefs about the positive and negative effects of worry and its controllability)	• "Worry helps me solve problems and prepare for the worst." • "If I worry, it means I really care, that I'm taking the situation seriously." • "If I don't stop worrying, I'm going to have a nervous breakdown." • "If I had more willpower, I could stop worrying."
5. *Additional Beliefs* (other beliefs I have about worry that do not fall into the categories above)	_____ _____ _____ _____

her from making a mistake and retiring from work too early. On the other hand, the worry was an "unstoppable force" that was robbing her of any present enjoyment. Any advantages of worry were outweighed by a mountain of misery and anxiety.

Worry Process Phase

Once an intrusive thought activates your underlying worry beliefs, the worry process can run on its own. As you saw in the cognitive model of worry diagram, four key features of the worry process perpetuate a downward spiral. When we begin to worry, there is a strong desire to stop the worry process—an effort to control the worry. There is also a search for relief, often by trying to obtain reassurance from others that everything will be all right. At the same time, we keep seeking solutions to the anticipated problem, and when we don't find one, we keep worrying—and then we start to worry about worrying and what it's doing to us. So let's take a closer look at these four elements of the worry process.

1. Effort to Control Worry

How many times have you heard people say, "Oh, don't worry about it" or "Stop worrying"? Of course that's the whole problem—you can't stop worrying. You want to retort, "Of course I know I should stop worrying, but I can't!" Interestingly, even though worriers know they can't control worry, that does not stop them from trying. It is well known that people prone to worry try hard not to worry.

> The harder you try to "not worry," the more you will worry.

Harvard psychologist Daniel Wegner discovered a phenomenon known as the *ironic effects of mental control*.[47] In his research he had individuals try not to think about something like a white bear for several minutes. After they stopped trying to suppress thoughts of a white bear, he discovered they had more thoughts about white bears intrude into their mind than the group of individuals that had not tried to suppress their thoughts. In other words, trying not to think about white bears caused people to think about white bears even more than if they had just left the thought alone.

Self-Help Exercise 11.1. Trying Not to Think about Something

Set a timer for 2 minutes and try to think about a white bear. Make a tick mark on a sheet of paper every time your mind wanders from the white bear. Now repeat the experiment, only this time try not to think about white bears for 2 minutes. **Make a tick mark every time the thought of a white bear intrudes into your mind.** Have a look at your tick marks. Did you have more tick marks when trying *not* to think about the white bear? Most people find it much harder to suppress a thought than to maintain their focus on a thought. Thought formation is much easier than thought prevention or dismissal.

The more you try not to worry, the more you worry: If you apply this phenomenon to the worry process, it's obvious that the more you try to stop worrying, the more you will worry. Given that worry focuses on issues that are really important to you, as opposed to a trivial thought like white bears, the paradoxical effects of intentional mental control will be even more pronounced.

A number of mental control strategies are known to make the worry process much worse:

- *Cognitive suppression* (telling yourself not to worry)

- *Self-reassurance* (telling yourself everything will be okay)

- *Reassurance from others* (asking family/friends if everything will be all right)

- *Checking* (engaging in some repetitive act to relieve doubt and uncertainty)

- *Punishment* (criticizing yourself for worrying)

- *Emotion suppression* (trying to suppress the distress and anxiety associated with worry)

Cognitive therapy targets these negative mental control efforts to reverse the downward spiral of the worry process.

2. Search for Relief

Most people with persistent and excessive worry will do almost anything to obtain some relief from the worry process and its associated anxiety. The worrier knows the best way to reduce anxiety is to believe that everything will be all right, so she seeks reassurance from others—"Do you think everything will be okay?"—or tries to convince herself that "everything will be okay" using clever arguments or trying to come up with solutions to convince herself she's prepared for the worst. But the problem with worry is that it's always about future events, and *no one can know the future.* So the desire for safety and certainty is futile. In fact, paradoxically, it contributes significantly to the persistence of worry.

There is a strong link between feeling anxious and worry. We believe that feeling anxious proves we *should* be worried. Ironically, we then assume the inverse is true: if I don't feel anxious, I don't have anything to worry about. Even though we might reduce anxiety by taking a tranquilizer, this can't change the future or ensure that what we're worried about will not in fact occur. The belief that feeling anxiety justi-fies worry (and that feeling calm alleviates the need to worry) is a good example of the thinking error of *emotional reasoning* discussed in Chapter 3.

Sylvia noticed that when she became stressed or overwhelmed with work demands she started to worry about her work performance ("I'm just throwing this report together; everyone will know it's not up to my standard" or "I'll never make these deadlines"). The more anxious she felt, the worse the worry, and the more she wor-ried, the worse the anxiety. On occasion she would take an Ativan and almost imme-diately feel less anxious and worried. But she didn't like taking medication; it made her less sharp at work, and she realized she was not learning how to deal effectively with her tendency to worry.

> We worry more because we feel anxious, and we feel anxious because we are worried! In cognitive therapy for worry we focus on breaking the link between worry and anxiety by addressing faulty emotional reasoning and discouraging the relentless search for relief.

3. Failed Problem Solving

Invariably, worry involves an incessant search for solutions—some way to deal with the predicted catastrophe that is the focus of worry. In his book *Anxiety Free,* Robert Leahy noted that needing an answer **right now** is an important contributor to wor-ry.[28] Research has shown that worriers can solve problems as well as nonworriers. However, worriers show other weaknesses in their approach to problem solving:

- Lack of confidence in their problem-solving ability
- Tendency to be overly focused on future threat
- Negative expectation about the problem-solving outcome
- Search for a perfect solution
- Tendency to focus on irrelevant information or compulsively check to reduce uncertainty[48]

The end result is that chronic worriers spend a lot of time "spinning their tires." They think through numerous possible responses to a feared outcome but end up rejecting each solution as unacceptable. This leaves them with a feeling of helplessness, unable to deal with an encroaching world of threat, danger, and uncertainty.

Derrick, age 35 and single, worried about the disapproval of others and rejection, especially when he dated. He would mentally run through various scenarios for how he could ensure that his date was attracted to him. He read numerous books on dating and even attended a few sessions with a dating coach, but in the end he rejected all the advice. Nothing seemed capable of guaranteeing a woman's approval and acceptance. And so he was left fretting, worrying about how he could overcome his anxiety about possible rejection.

4. Worry about Worry

British psychologist Adrian Wells is a leading expert on the psychology of worry. He introduced the concept of "worry about worry" and has found that this type of worry (called "meta-worry") is a major contributor to the persistence of pathological worry and GAD.[49] The person who "worries about worrying" holds a set of negative beliefs about worry: "I will go crazy unless I stop worrying," "I have lost all control over worry," "I can't do anything productive as long as I am worrying." Once individuals become worried about their chronic worry, they enter a whole new level of pathological worry. This is because your "fear of worry" will cause you to try even harder to control it and to suppress any unwanted thoughts and feelings. Avoidance and the search for safety take on a renewed sense of urgency as the person is convinced he must do whatever it takes to avoid the experience of anxiety or worry.

> The worry process sustains its own momentum because of efforts to control worry, search for relief, failed problem solving, and worry about worry, each of which is targeted by cognitive therapy.

After years of worry, Sylvia was convinced that her life had been ruined by her pathological worry. She came to fear the worry episodes and tried to figure out her worry triggers so she could avoid these situations or experiences. Of course this turned out to be futile and only left her feeling trapped and defeated.

Your Worry Profile

Although all chronic worry generally shares the characteristics described above, everyone has a unique worry profile. As the anxiety profile you developed in Chapter 5 helped you construct a cognitive therapy program uniquely for you, your worry profile will guide your cognitive therapy specifically for worry. The following steps will help you build your worry profile.

Step 1: Identify Worry Concerns

Begin by identifying one to three main worry concerns or issues that have dominated your thinking recently—choose those that occur most frequently or are most distressing, if you have many. Reviewing Worksheet 11.1 can remind you what your main worry concerns are. Then start learning more about those worries by recording your worry experiences in a diary. Many of our clients find this exercise not only gives them new insights into their worrying but is actually therapeutic because it helps to bring some order and perspective to the worry process.

Self-Help Exercise 11.2. Monitoring Your Worry Episodes

If you have intense and daily worry, record your worry episodes on Worksheet 11.4 for one week. If your worry is less frequent, monitor your worry over a 2- to 3-week period. Try to capture the initial triggers—the situations and the anxious intrusive thought that caused you to start worrying. In the worry content column, describe the possible threatening or distressing situation that is the focus of your worry. Mark with an asterisk the worries that relate to the main worry concerns you listed in Worksheet 11.1. Are these worry concerns happening more or less frequently than you expected? Are the worries you noted in Worksheet 11.1 still the main problem for you, or is there a new issue you should be targeting for treatment? Next record the approximate length of the episode and your level of distress or anxiety while worrying. Finally, write down how you tried to stop worrying. What did you do to reduce your anxiety or stop yourself from worrying? Was it effective?

Step 2: Recognize the Catastrophe

Worry always focuses on the possibility of future threat and danger. We tend to *hope* for positive future events or good fortune; we *worry* over the possibility of bad outcomes. Thus chronic pathological worry is characterized by an overwhelming preoccupation with catastrophic thinking. Worriers focus almost exclusively on the worst possible outcome, exaggerating its probability: "I am definitely going to fail this course, and then I'll have to quit school."

Self-Help Exercise 11.3. Tracking Your Catastrophic Thinking

Over the next week or two, use Worksheet 6.2 to track your catastrophic thinking *during* worry episodes. While you're worrying, focus on the future negative circumstance or threatening outcome you fear might occur. Write

Worry Diary

Instructions: Write down significant worry episodes. Try to complete the form as close to the worry episode as possible to increase the accuracy of your remarks.

Date and Time of Day	Initial Trigger What did you hear or what thought crossed your mind that got you worrying?	Worry Content What were you worrying about? Briefly describe. Put an asterisk beside those that relate to your main worry concerns listed in Worksheet 11.1.	Duration of Worry (minutes or hours)	Distress Level during Worrying (0–100)	Control Attempts What did you do to stop worrying? Was it successful?

Reprinted with permission from *Cognitive Therapy of Anxiety Disorders* by David A. Clark and Aaron T. Beck (p. 442). Copyright 2010 by The Guilford Press.

down your beliefs about the likelihood and severity of the outcome and about your ability to cope. Also, are there any safety aspects to the situation that you are overlooking?

When Sylvia did this exercise, she discovered that whenever she worried about her husband's health she was thinking he would have a heart attack, die, and then she would be left to live out the rest of her life in loneliness and despair. When worrying, she rated the probability of his heart attack as very high (80/100). When she wasn't worried and anxious about his health, her probability estimate dropped to 20%. Sylvia was able to recognize that her tendency to exaggerate the probability of bad outcomes only made her anxiety and worry much worse.

Step 3: Discover Worry Beliefs

Because the way you evaluate your worry plays an important role in its persistence and uncontrollability, it's important to discover how you think about being worried with all of life's cares. What do you think is so awful or bad for you about having this worry episode? What do you think might be positive or beneficial for you about engaging in worry? Go back to Table 11.2 and place an asterisk beside the two or three negative beliefs that are most relevant to your worry. Then, on a separate sheet of paper, write down three or four positive beliefs you may hold about your worry—that it will help you solve problems, prepare for the worst, stay focused, stay motivated to act, and so forth. Most chronic worriers believe there is a positive function of worry and therefore are reluctant to give up worry entirely, even though it is severely distressing.

Self-Help Exercise 11.4. Recording Your Beliefs about Worry

One of the best ways to identify the underlying beliefs that drive your chronic worry is to record your thoughts while you're worrying. **Use Worksheet 11.5 to record your positive and negative thoughts about worry during worry episodes.**

Sylvia found during this exercise that a number of beliefs about worry were activated during her worry episodes. Her most dominant negative beliefs were "I can't

Monitoring Your Worry Beliefs

Instructions: This form should be completed during episodes of daily worry. Try to complete the form as close to the worry episode as possible to increase the accuracy of your remarks.

Date and Duration of Worry	**Primary Worry Concern** Focus on the worry concerns listed in Worksheet 11.1 or a new recurring worry discovered from Worksheet 11.4. State the worry, including the worst outcome you are thinking.	**Negative Thoughts (Beliefs) about the Worry Episode** What do you think is so awful or bad for you about having this worry episode?	**Positive Thoughts (Beliefs) about the Worry Episode** What do you think might be positive or beneficial for you about having this worry episode?	**Extent of Worry about Worrying** (0–100*)

*Rate extent of "worry about worrying" associated with present episode from 0 ("not at all worried that I am worrying") to 100 ("extremely worried that I had another worry episode").

The activation of your beliefs about worry will lead to various automatic thoughts during worry episodes, and dealing with these thoughts and beliefs about worry is an important part of the cognitive therapy approach.

get anything done while I am worrying," "The worry is causing so much stress that I could have a heart attack," and "If I don't control this worry, the anxiety will become unbearable." Her positive beliefs were "Worry keeps me focused," "Sometimes I see my way through a problem because of worry," and "Worry ensures that I am prepared for the worst in the future."

Step 4: Specify Control and Safety Strategies

A final component of your worry profile involves identifying the worry control strategies and safety behaviors that you may have come to rely on to manage chronic worry. Go back to page 247 and place an asterisk beside the mental control strategies that you rely on most often in your attempts to prevent or at least reduce worry. Also review how you filled out Worksheets 5.6 and 5.7 and again note which behavioral and cognitive strategies you use most often in the context of worry. Don't forget to include repeated attempts at problem solving, reassurance seeking, and any repeated checking strategies you may use in a search for safety and a sense of certainty about the future.

Self-Help Exercise 11.5.
Creating Your Worry Profile

Use Worksheet 11.6 to compile all the aspects of your persistent and uncontrollable worry. You will use your Worry Profile form to customize your worry rehabilitation plan based on the treatment strategies discussed in the rest of the chapter.

Cognitive Treatment for Worry

Step 1: Determine Your Worry Type

Worry can be classified along two dimensions: realistic versus imagined problems and productive versus unproductive consequences. This produces four types of repetitive thought.

Worry Profile

Instructions: Complete this form by reviewing your responses to the four steps of worry assessment discussed in this section of the chapter.

Step 1. Worry Triggers

a. Personal goals, values, and concerns related to worry: _____

_____

b. Initial unwanted intrusive thoughts: _____

_____

Step 2. Catastrophic Thinking (while worrying)

a. Estimated likelihood: _____

b. Assumed severity: _____

c. Perceived ability to cope: _____

Step 3. Worry Beliefs

a. Negative beliefs about worry: _____

_____

b. Positive beliefs about worry: _____

_____

Step 4. Control and Safety Strategies

a. Worry control strategies: _____

_____

b. Safety search strategies (i.e., how you try to attain a sense of calm, assurance, and certainty):

_____

Realistic, Productive Problem Solving	Imagined, Productive Thoughtful Planning
Realistic but Unproductive Worry	Imagined Unproductive Worry

The first cell, realistic, productive problem solving, is a type of repetitive thought that leads to highly effective solutions. Thoughtful planning about imagined outcomes occurs when we think more constructively about possible responses to hypothetical future difficulties (such as developing an emergency plan for a house fire). Cognitive therapy focuses on the bottom two cells, unproductive realistic or imagined worry. The goal of treatment is to change unproductive worry into the more productive, solution-based thinking shown in the top two cells.

Not all worry is about imagined or hypothetical possibilities in the future. Sometimes we worry about real events that are unfolding in our daily lives. You might be facing treatment for a serious illness and be worried about the outcome, or you may have lost your job and be having difficulty finding new employment, or you may be having serious arguments with your spouse and be worried about a breakup. **The first step in cognitive therapy is to determine whether the worry is about a realistic problem or an imagined ("what if") situation.** Jerry had missed three mortgage payments in the last 9 months, and she was now getting calls from collection agencies about missed credit card payments. Jerry was worried sick about her financial situation and the possibility that she might have to declare bankruptcy and could lose her house to foreclosure. Jerry's situation looked desperate, and so her anxiety and worry about finances seemed reasonable.

Brian, on the other hand, was a 33-year-old radiologist who had just joined the diagnostic neuroimaging unit of a local hospital. Despite comments from the chief radiologist that his diagnostic work was good, Brian felt constantly worried that he might make a mistake in reading a scan and that he was not being as productive as the other radiologists. When he looked at his billing figures in comparison to the other radiologists, he saw that he was within an acceptable range of his colleagues. But Brian could never be the most productive radiologist because he was slower and kept rechecking his diagnostic reports to ensure he was not misdiagnosing a scan. In Brian's case his worries "What if I misdiagnose a patient?" and "What if I fall behind my colleagues in productivity?" were imagined threats (i.e., they weren't happening but potentially could happen).

Whether your worry is about an immediate realistic problem or an imagined threat (a "what if"), you need to ask yourself whether your worry is productive or unproductive. Jerry's worry about bankruptcy was realistic, but was her worry productive? Did it lead to action that would solve her problem, or was it unproductive in interfering in her problem-solving ability? Brian's imagined threat of job failure was more clearly unproductive in that it caused him to check and recheck his diagnostic decisions, thereby reducing his work efficiency and productivity. Do your worry episodes move you closer to your life goals, or have they become a barrier, robbing you of life enjoyment and satisfaction?

Self-Help Exercise 11.6.
Determining Whether Your Worry Is Productive or Unproductive

First determine whether your worry focuses on an immediate, realistic problem or a more distant, hypothetical negative situation (a "what if"). Next consider the positive and negative consequences of worry to determine whether it is mainly productive or unproductive. (You can look back at Table 11.1 if you're not sure.) Use Worksheet 11.7 to record your findings. If you're not sure of the consequences of worry, monitor your worry episodes and record the immediate effects of worry or ask your therapist, a close friend, or a family member for input on how worry affects you. Repeat this exercise for each worry concern listed in Worksheet 11.1 or recorded in your Worry Diary (Worksheet 11.4).

⋛ Troubleshooting Tips ⋚

You may have difficulty knowing whether a worry is about imagined or realistic problems. If there is already concrete evidence in your life that the problem you worry about is developing, then the worry is more realistic. For example, worrying that your teenage son could be arrested for a serious crime would be realistic if he is already committing minor crimes. Imagined worries, in contrast, deal with possible bad outcomes where there is currently no evidence that your life is moving in this direction. For example, being worried about cancer would be imagined if there are no medical indications that you might have cancer at this time. So imagined worries are developments that can happen but for which there is no realistic evidence these problems are presently unfolding in your life.

Step 2: Use Constructive Problem Solving for Realistic Worry

Does your worry involve an immediate, realistic concern, such as an impending divorce, one-year follow-up after cancer treatment, a difficult teenager who is fail-

Consequences of Worry

Instructions: Write down one of your main worries from Worksheet 11.1 or your Worry Diary (Worksheet 11.4) and then list some of the positive and negative consequences of worrying about this concern. After listing your worry consequences, review them and decide whether your worry is mainly productive or unproductive. Make a copy of this form so you can repeat the exercise if you have more than one worry concern.

1. Main worry concern: _____

_____

_____

2. Negative consequences of worry:

    a. _____

    b. _____

    c. _____

    d. _____

    e. _____

3. Positive consequences of worry:

    a. _____

    b. _____

    c. _____

    d. _____

    e. _____

4. Overall, my worry on this topic is productive.   Yes   No

5. Overall, my worry on this topic is unproductive.   Yes   No

ing in school, unemployment, or bank foreclosure? If so, try constructive problem solving
as described by Robert Leahy in his book *The
Worry Cure*.[48]

Before you can do any constructive problem solving for a realistic concern, you have to
figure out how much responsibility and control
you have over the outcome of the problem. You
will have almost 100% control over some problems, such as noticing that you are low on gas
or that you need to leave home sooner because
you are consistently late for work. Other problems you may have only partial control and

The first step in cognitive therapy for
worry is to identify whether your worry
focuses on a realistic or more imagined
("what if") problem. If the worry
concern deals with a more immediate,
realistic problem, then *constructive
problem solving* is the main therapeutic
approach. The other strategies that
follow are more relevant for worry
about imagined problems ("what if").

responsibility for, such as being selected for job promotion, dealing with marital conflict, reducing your risk of a heart attack, or improving your return on investments.
You may have little or no control over other problems such as the results of a test for
cancer, your spouse's chronic medical illness, or the recent death of a loved one.

Having an accurate assessment of your control over and responsibility for a
problem is a key aspect of productive worry. Overestimating how much control and
responsibility you have causes anxiety and stress; underestimating can lead to paraly-
sis and inactivity. The Control Pie Chart in Worksheet 11.8 can be used to develop a
healthier perspective on your role in the problematic situations that worry you.

Sylvia filled in a Control Pie Chart for her worry about getting housework done.
At first she assumed that housework was 100% under her control. But filling in
the control chart revealed that other factors—whether she had to work late (20%),
whether her husband messed up the house (15%), whether the housekeeper showed

Repeatedly using the Control
Pie Chart whenever you worry
can help you learn the important
difference between what can
and cannot be controlled—a line
that is often blurred for chronic
worriers. Once you identify those
boundaries, you can tackle solving
problems under your control but
learn to accept those that are not.

up for her weekly clean (10%), and whether the dog
had had a particularly bad week (5%)—affected her
control. In reality Sylvia had only 50% control over
keeping the house clean. Once she realized this, Sylvia was able to use constructive problem solving to
deal with her 50% of the responsibility, but she also
had to learn to accept the possibility of an unclean
house due to the 50% outside her control.

Once you've accepted a more realistic view of
your responsibility in a worry issue, you can use the
following problem-solving steps to deal with that
part of the concern that is under your control.

1. Identify the problem.

2. Brainstorm possible solutions.

Control Pie Chart

Instructions: Identify a single worry concern that has immediate, realistic negative outcomes. Next write down all of the factors that can influence the outcome of this situation (e.g., other people's actions, your actions, the environment, or the situation). After determining the various causes or influences on the problem, assign percentages to reflect the amount of responsibility and control each factor has on the problem outcome. All of these influences should add up to 100%. What percentage of control over this problem did you assign to yourself?

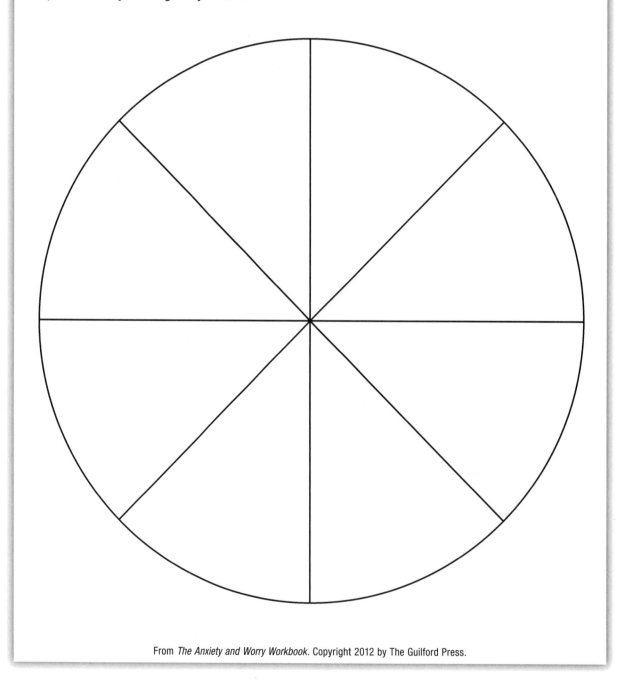

3. Evaluate each solution.

4. Develop a solution-based action plan.

5. Evaluate the outcome of the action plan.

Identifying the problem starts with figuring out what part of the problem you control. Joanne was worried that she might not get the promotion she had applied for at work. The Control Pie Chart showed that she had only 60% control over the outcome and that the only thing she could control was her preparation for the promotion interview. So preparing herself for the interview became the identified problem. Joanne brainstormed a number of ways to prepare for the interview:

■ Write out a short, clear explanation of her past experiences, skills, and what she would do in the new position if promoted.

■ Talk to a couple of colleagues who had recently been promoted through an interview process.

■ Write down a list of possible interview questions and prepare potential responses.

■ Do "mock interviews" with a coworker.

■ Discuss the promotion interview with her supervisor.

■ Confide in her husband about her anxiety over the selection interview.

■ Seek tranquilizers from her family physician.

Next Joanne evaluated each of the brainstorming solutions. She decided that the first four options were the most constructive solutions and would do most for preparing her for the interview. Each of the last three options had serious drawbacks, so she decided to eliminate them. Based on the acceptable brainstorming solutions, Joanne developed the following action plan:

> Remember the goal with problem solving is to lower your anxiety and deal more effectively with the problem situation. Unfortunately, it cannot guarantee a desired outcome.

I will take 30 minutes each evening (Monday–Friday) over the next 2 weeks and work on preparing for the promotion interview. I will begin by writing out a five-page explanation of my past experiences, skills, and vision for the new position. I'll read this over several times to familiarize myself with my explanation. I'll include a list of possible interview questions, including some possible questions that might focus on "gaps" in my résumé. I'll ask Larry and Meredith about the interview process since they were recently promoted. I'll approach Judy, my closest friend at work, to do two mock interviews at least 3 days before the actual interview. I'll get her feedback on my performance and make adjustments where needed.

At first Joanne thought the best way to evaluate the success of her action plan was by whether or not she got the job promotion. But then she realized this was not the appropriate outcome because only 60% of the outcome was under her influence. Whether she got the promotion depended on the qualifications of the other candidates and the decision making of the selection committee. So she decided to evaluate the success of the action plan on whether it reduced her feelings of anxiety and worry over the interview. She tracked her anxiety level and worry using the Worry Diary (Worksheet 11.4) and noticed that the frequency and intensity of her worry episodes dropped after she implemented her action plan.

Self-Help Exercise 11.7.
Practicing Constructive Problem Solving

Practice the constructive problem-solving approach with a problem that concerns you. You may want to start with a fairly easy problem that is only a mild concern to you (e.g., how to keep my car clean, how to get to work on time more consistently, how to get along better with my roommate). After you've mastered the problem-solving approach with these situations, move on to one of your main worry concerns. Schedule specific time periods to work on your constructive problem-solving plan. Develop an action plan, implement it, and then evaluate its effect on your level of worry and anxiety.

⋛ Troubleshooting Tips ⋚

If you tried constructive problem solving and it didn't help with your anxiety and worry, make sure one or more of the following did not undermine your efforts.

■ *Seeking perfect solutions*—rejecting every response to a problem because it didn't provide a perfect solution.

■ *Overestimating your control*—thinking you can ensure a desired outcome when you have only partial control or influence over the outcome.

■ *Unrealistic expectations*—constructive problem solving will only reduce worry and anxiety; it won't eliminate it entirely.

- *Vague action plan*—you must be very specific about your action plan: what to do, how to do it, and when to do it.

- *Inadequate brainstorming*—it is important to generate a list of several options to a problem before you start eliminating them as inappropriate.

- *Highly "imagined" threat*—constructive problem solving cannot deal with vague, remote, and highly imagined or hypothetical threats that have only limited connection with reality ("What if I die young?" or "What if no one likes me?" or "What if I never succeed in life?").

Step 3: Correct Catastrophic Thinking

In the cognitive model of worry (see the diagram on page 241), catastrophic thinking is always at the heart of unproductive and excessive worry. The activation of negative beliefs about threat and helplessness causes us to focus almost exclusively on future threat and danger. *Worry feeds on catastrophic thinking!* If you stop catastrophizing, you will cut off the life supply for worry. This is easier said than done, since catastrophizing is second nature for chronic worriers. But we've found that teaching chronic worriers "how to kick the catastrophizing habit" can bring relief from excessive and unproductive worry.

The evidence gathering, error identification, alternative generation, and decatastrophizing strategies discussed in Chapter 6 can be used to reduce worry. First review your Worry Profile (Worksheet 11.6), focusing on how you overestimate the likelihood and severity of a worry-related future threat and underestimate your ability to cope with this threat. These three elements (likelihood, severity, and perceived coping) represent the core elements of catastrophic thinking. Use Worksheet 6.3 to gather evidence that you are overestimating the likelihood and severity of an imagined negative outcome. Then identify the cognitive errors in your thinking (see Chapter 3) and work on generating a more probable, realistic perspective on the worry concern.

Sylvia was very worried about her husband's health. Richard had recently been diagnosed with unstable angina. Her worry was based on catastrophic thinking; she was convinced he could have a fatal heart attack at any moment and that she would be left a lonely, grief-stricken widow. Sylvia began by determining whether she was overestimating the likelihood that unstable angina automatically leads to a fatal heart attack. She looked up information on unstable angina and learned that it is a common condition associated with increased risk for heart attack. She obtained medical information indicating that the average risk for a heart attack in a single month is approximately 10% or less and fewer than 5% die from heart attack due to unstable angina in the same time period. She also learned that various medications and lifestyle changes can reduce the probability of heart attack in unstable angina. Based on this evidence,

Use evidence gathering, error identification, and generation of alternative perspectives to correct the tendency to exaggerate the probability and severity of threat in chronic worry.

Sylvia could see that she was exaggerating the probability of her husband's having a heart attack and underestimating the various medical, dietary, and activity-based interventions that would lower his risk. In addition, she realized she was jumping to conclusions and had tunnel vision when thinking about her husband's condition. Sylvia came up with the following alternative perspective.

Richard has a chronic medical condition that places him at increased risk of a fatal heart attack. Millions of Americans live long and productive lives with this condition. Although Richard has an elevated risk of heart attack, his chances of survival at any given moment greatly outweigh his chances of death. There are many medical interventions, medications, and lifestyle changes that can effectively lower (but not eliminate) Richard's risk of a heart attack. Like so many others, we can learn to live many years with this health threat.

Sylvia implemented her new perspective every time she started to worry about Richard's health; she reminded herself of the evidence for the more realistic alternative and the evidence against the catastrophic assumption that Richard would die at any moment from a heart attack.

Self-Help Exercise 11.8.
Developing an Alternative to Catastrophic Thinking

Complete an evidence-gathering form (Worksheet 6.3) and develop an alternative perspective (Worksheet 6.5) that challenges your catastrophic thinking about a particular worry concern. Review these forms and add to them each time you experience a worry episode. After repeated experience you will become more skilled at correcting your initial catastrophic thinking earlier and earlier in the worry process.

⋛ Troubleshooting Tips ⋚

If correcting your catastrophic thinking through evidence gathering does not reduce your worry, you may be using evidence to reassure yourself that the worst won't happen. Make sure you're using evidence gathering *only to correct your biased estimates of threat probability and severity.* Remember that you can't predict the future and bad things could happen (Richard *could* have a fatal heart attack) and that evidence gathering is not a "magic cure." You won't automatically stop worrying by reminding yourself of the evidence. Instead, evidence gathering will gradually help lower worry because you'll be engaged in numerous repeated corrections of biased catastrophic thinking.

Step 4: Face the Worst

There is always some dreaded catastrophe, a worst-case scenario that we don't want to think about when worried. Thomas Borkovec, a pioneer in worry research and a professor of psychology at Penn State University, has argued that we worry to avoid some dreaded future threat or danger.[50] For example, a father might worry about why his teenage son is late coming home on a weekend night rather than imagine he has been in a tragic car accident. A person might worry about the results of a diagnostic medical test rather than think about living with cancer. Or an individual might worry about whether she has offended a close friend rather than think about losing that friendship. In other words, worry is often an attempt to avoid thinking about some dreaded ultimate catastrophe. The problem is that worry is not an effective avoidance strategy and is one of the reasons for the persistence of generalized anxiety. Doing the opposite of avoidance, *facing your worst fear,* has become an important step in cognitive therapy for worry.

> Repeatedly exposing yourself to your most extreme worry fears is a useful therapy approach for challenging core beliefs that maintain worry, such as that having your worst fear come true would be unbearable and that you would be completely helpless and overwhelmed by the experience.

Self-Help Exercise 11.9.
Exposing Yourself to Worry—and Then Decatastrophizing

You can learn to face your worst fear by starting with a *worry catastrophe story.* **Take a worry concern and ask yourself, "What is the worst possible outcome, the ultimate catastrophe, that I fear most?"** If you are worried about a relationship, it might be fear of losing that relationship; if you have financial worries, it might be losing everything and declaring bankruptcy; if it's worries about work, it might be losing your job and being chronically unemployed. Use Worksheet 11.9 to write out a description of the worst imagined outcome to the worry concern. Don't write down what you think might happen. Instead, use your imagination and write down the worst outcome, the worst catastrophe, you can imagine.

Once you have developed your worry catastrophe account, you're ready to engage in *directed worry expression*. **Set aside 30–45 minutes each day as your time to worry.** Find a quiet, private place where you can let yourself be anxious and worried. During this time, verbally express your worries, talk out loud, repeating your worries over and over. Don't try to suppress your worries; do the opposite—express your worries. Read your worry catastrophe story aloud, really concentrating on it and getting yourself into the story as much as possible. What you are doing with this exercise is facing your worries and worst fears. Of course, as with all exposure, it is important that you do this over and over again, repeatedly every day for 2–3 weeks. If you find yourself worrying about something during the day, write down the worry so you can use it later during your scheduled worry expression period. Remind yourself, "I don't have to worry about this now; I want to save this worry for my worry session this evening." Do this exercise until you feel minimal anxiety or distress when thinking about the worst possible outcome associated with your worry.

A final step in "facing your worst fear" is to write out a *decatastrophizing plan*. In reality, how would you cope with experiencing your worst fear? How would you learn to live with cancer, live on your own, or deal with the loss of your dream job? What would you do if you found out your spouse was having an affair or that your teenage son was arrested on a drug charge? **Write down practical, realistic, concrete steps you would take to deal with this catastrophe in your life.** You could consider this your emergency plan— what you would do if the very worst happened. You can think about this as similar to creating an emergency response strategy for house fires. We don't plan on our house burning down, but it's a good idea to know what to do in case it happens. The same is true with your worry-related worst fear. It may never happen, but it is good idea to have a plan. Might you be able to deal with the catastrophe better than you think? You could seek out information on the catastrophe, how others have dealt with it, and incorporate this into your decatastrophizing plan.

Sylvia began by writing down all her worries about retirement and a worst-case scenario that involved a plummet in her pension income. She wrote out what it would

Your Worst Fear

Instructions: Write out in as much detail as possible (250–500 words) what it would be like to live the worst fear related to your worry concern. What might happen to bring about the worst outcome? How would it affect you physically, emotionally, behaviorally, and socially? How would you respond to this catastrophic outcome? How would you try to cope? Would it be effective? How would your life change if you lived out the catastrophe? How would friends and family treat you after you experienced the worst fear? Would they abandon you? What would be the long-term effects of experiencing the catastrophe?

_____

_____

_____

_____

_____

_____

_____

_____

_____

_____

_____

(Use extra pages to complete your worry catastrophe story.)

feel like to be "broke" and have to watch her expenses. Sylvia imagined how her friends and adult children might react and what life would be like with little money. Then she scheduled 30 minutes each day when she read aloud all her worries about retirement and the worst-case scenario. She tried to imagine as vividly as possible what it would be like to be a "financially strapped senior on a fixed income." She faithfully completed the worry expression exercise for 23 consecutive days until she felt bored and disinterested in the exercise. At this point she was able to reexamine the retirement situation and write out a decatastrophizing plan—how she would deal with a sudden loss of investment income during retirement. She discovered that she would be able to cope with this situation much better than she had imagined.

≥ Troubleshooting Tips ≤

If facing your worst fear does not help reduce your worry, make sure you're dealing with "the worst possible outcome" related to your worry. The exercise won't help if you tone down the imagined outcome, making it less fearsome or anxiety provoking. The worst fear has to be very extreme. And you have to write down your worries and the worst-case scenario. You can't just rely on your memory. Also you need to read it out loud over and over. Finally, you have to do this exercise again and again. Repetition is critical! Many people try this once or twice and then conclude it doesn't work. Directed worry expression won't be effective if you do it a couple of times; you have to do it so often that you actually begin to feel bored and disinterested.

Step 5: Reformat Worry Beliefs

Often it's difficult to make progress on worry until the underlying beliefs about the worry process are identified and corrected. Refer back to Worksheet 11.5 to review the positive and negative beliefs that might characterize your worry. You can use the evidence gathering, cost–benefit analysis, and generating alternatives strategies discussed in Chapter 6 to correct these worry beliefs. Focus on the main beliefs outlined in your worry profile (Worksheet 11.6).

Jason, a senior in college, worried constantly about his GPA. He believed that worrying made him study more, but also that worry was causing so much anxiety and stress that it probably interfered with his performance on tests. He came to fear worry and tried to control it, but with little success. Jason examined evidence from past experience to challenge these beliefs and was surprised to discover that worry did not have as much effect on his test scores as he thought; nor did it act as a

Correcting maladaptive worry beliefs is also an effective intervention for reducing worry about worry (worrying about the negative consequences of being a worrier).

good motivator for studying. He realized he had been overgeneralizing from a couple of times when worry seemed to affect his test grade. So he came up with an alternative view that a certain amount of worry about exams was normal and could actually be productive. What he needed to work on was excessive worry. Whenever he started to fret that worry would cause him to do poorly on an exam, Jason would stop, engage in 20 minutes of directed worry expression, and then resume studying. This exercise helped to correct his distorted belief about the negative effects of worry.

Self-Help Exercise 11.10.
Correcting Negative Beliefs about Worry

Take 30 minutes twice a week to work on correcting maladaptive beliefs about worry. Use evidence gathering, cost–benefit analysis, and generating alternatives to correct your positive and negative beliefs about worry. During worry episodes, review your evidence gathering and cost–benefit sheets to counter the automatic maladaptive worry beliefs. Conclude this exercise with an actual response that is more consistent with your corrected worry beliefs.

Step 6: Surrender Control

Earlier in the chapter we discussed the fact that the harder you try to control worry, the worse it gets. So it is important to identify your worry control responses and then work on eliminating worry control from your life.

Sylvia identified three ways that she tried to control worry. She would constantly tell herself to stop worrying (cognitive suppression), try to reassure herself that things will turn out fine (self-reassurance), and ask others whether they thought her feared outcome wouldn't happen (reassurance seeking from others). Of course, none of these control efforts worked, so she kept on worrying. Sylvia used four approaches to reduce her worry control efforts.

Self-Help Exercise 11.11.
Substituting New Strategies for Old Worry Control Responses

Take 2 weeks and work specifically on worry control. Try to catch yourself engaging in the worry control strategies listed in your worry profile (Worksheet 11.6). Practice using the four strategies described below instead of the old worry control responses. After 2 weeks, evaluate whether you've made any progress in adopting a more "accepting attitude" toward worry.

■ *Accept worry.* Surrendering control means that you accept the worry process. Rather than fight worry, you "ride through" the worry episodes. If you brain decides to worry, let it. Allow the worry thoughts to float through your mind. You might even want to take the view of an observer, watching the worry thoughts go through your mind as if you were a bystander watching a parade. Come to view worry as a *normal process* that does not need to interfere in your life or rob you of enjoyment. In *The Worry Cure*[48] Robert Leahy discusses the importance of acceptance in reducing the tendency to worry.

■ *Suspend worry.* When you have a worry episode, write down your concern and then save it for your scheduled worry expression period. Remind yourself, "This is a good point; I'll write this down and make sure I spend lots of time worrying about this issue later this evening, during my worry expression period." At first you might find it hard to wait, but keep practicing and eventually you'll master the ability to hold off on worry until later.

■ *Normalize worry.* Work on normalizing worry episodes by continuing with your daily activities to the best of your ability. If you can't concentrate because of worry, engage in simpler, more routine tasks during worry episodes (clean the house, wash the car, reorganize your office, call a friend, etc.). What you want to avoid is stopping all activities to worry. This should occur only during the worry expression period. Engaging in life activities during worry episodes may also provide some natural distraction from the worry process.

■ *Prevent response control.* Once you have identified your most common worry control strategies, stop engaging in them. For example, you can stop asking other people for reassurance about the future (it's rather useless because they can't forecast the future any better than you!). You can also stop yourself from checking and rechecking to ensure everything is okay, and you can work on reducing your habit to overanalyze (overthink) an issue in order to reassure yourself.

> ⩣ **Troubleshooting Tips** ⩤
>
> You may find it difficult to reduce your worry control efforts. You may be tempted to give up after a few days. Remember, "old habits die hard," and it will take time to work on your natural tendency to control worry. Writing down your worry concerns, challenging your exaggerated thinking about future threats, saving your concerns for worry expression, and normalizing worry by maintaining engagement in your daily activities are the best strategies for reducing worry control. Remind yourself about the "white bear" (Self-Help Exercise 11.1): *the harder you try to control your worry, the worse it gets.*

Trying too hard to control worry (overcontrol) is the major problem in chronic worry rather than the opposite—having poor control over worry (undercontrol). This is why learning to let go of control and accepting anxiety are critical goals in cognitive therapy of worry.

Step 7: Accept Uncertainty

The final step in cognitive therapy for worry focuses on the issue of uncertainty. Canadian psychologist Michel Dugas has shown that difficulty accepting uncertainty is a key feature of generalized anxiety and worry[51]; that is, people worry to reassure themselves about the future. They are trying to reduce an uncertainty about the future by "thinking through" what is most likely to happen. Brodie, for example, was worried about his final exam in organic chemistry. He kept thinking about the prospects of failure, whether he was likely to fail, in an effort to convince himself of the likely outcome. Judy was worried about selling her house and kept thinking over and over whether she would ever find a buyer. Samantha worried that her husband might be having an affair and spent many hours trying to convince herself he was faithful and would not leave her. In each of these cases, the worry process is driven by a desire to "know the future," to reduce uncertainty. Most worriers will tell you they would rather know something bad is going to happen than to live with "not knowing."

The problem with the "need to know" is the future can never be known with absolute certainty. Worry is an attempt to reassure ourselves of the future—an attempt to reduce life's uncertainties, to eliminate the *what if*s in our life. But psychological research has found that this search for relief from uncertainty has the opposite effect; it makes us more anxious and worried about the future. Learning to accept risk and uncertainty will reduce worry and generalized anxiety.[52]

Self-Help Exercise 11.12.
Building Tolerance for Risk and Uncertainty

Work on your acceptance of uncertainty by taking one week to learn how you are struggling against uncertainty. **Complete Worksheet 11.10 during each worry episode to focus on the intolerance of uncertainty. Then in the second week review the worksheet and do a cost–benefit analysis of the advantages and disadvantages of accepting that future outcomes are uncertain (use Worksheet 6.4).** Are you convinced of the advantages of accepting uncertainty? Next repeatedly and intentionally focus on the possibility of the dreaded outcome associated with the worry until you feel less anxious about it (decatastrophize). **In fact, flood yourself with uncertainty thoughts.** Don't try to avoid or suppress them. Face the uncertainty head on and accept it. **Practice evaluating and correcting the uncertainty thinking associated with your worry. Finally, in the third week, expose yourself to uncertainty daily.** Try to do one or two activities each day that are different, more spontaneous, and associated with increased levels of uncertainty. The goal is to build up your tolerance and acceptance of risk and uncertainty.

Brodie reminded himself there is no such thing as a sure exam grade. He can't know what questions will be on the exam so he is forced to accept uncertainty. Being a student means living with the uncertainty of exams and their outcome. Focusing on exam uncertainty rather than trying to avoid it through reassurance seeking was an important step in reducing Brodie's worry.

One of the most effective ways to improve your acceptance of uncertainty is to practice exposing yourself to uncertainty in your daily life.[51] You can intentionally focus on the uncertainty in your daily activities. All of Sylvia's worry centered on the uncertainty of retirement, her husband's health, whether her son would find a job, and so on. She was convinced that she had to try to know the future, know how everything would turn out. Her worry focused on trying to eliminate negative outcomes and to reassure herself that "everything will be all right." For a self-help exercise, Sylvia's cognitive therapist had her rate the level of uncertainty associated with "non-worry" daily activities. For example, Sylvia noted that she took trips, drove places, attended meetings, and yet tolerated a level of uncertainty associated with them. The therapist then encouraged Sylvia to increase risk and uncertainty in her life. Some of her assignments included going to a new location in her city without taking her GPS, letting a friend drive the car rather than herself, reducing her preparation for a meeting at work, booking a short vacation trip on the spur of the moment, and inviting a

Risk and Uncertainty Record

Dates: from: _____ to: _____

Instructions: This form should be completed during episodes of daily worry. Try to complete the form as close to the worry episode as possible to increase the accuracy of your remarks.

Date and Duration of Worry	Primary Worry Concern Briefly describe your worries from Worksheets 11.1 and 11.4, including the worst outcome you are thinking.	Sequence of "What If" Questions List the "what if" questions that are generated during the worry episode.	Level of Uncertainty (0–100*)	Responses to Uncertainty What makes the uncertainty of this worry concern intolerable? How have you tried to reduce the uncertainty?

*Rate how much this worry makes you feel uncomfortably uncertain about the future outcome of this worry concern from 0 ("no feeling of uncertainty") to 100 ("I am feeling extremely tentative, uncertain about the outcome").

Reprinted with permission from *Cognitive Therapy of Anxiety Disorders* by David A. Clark and Aaron T. Beck (p. 445). Copyright 2010 by The Guilford Press.

273

Learning to accept the uncertainties of life and to live with "reasonable risk" is an important goal for overcoming excessive and unproductive worry.

new work colleague to dinner on short notice. All of these activities were designed to increase Sylvia's tolerance of risk and uncertainty. Of course, they also increased the level of spontaneity in her life. The net result was that Sylvia's anxiety and worry decreased as she learned to accept the uncertainties of life.

⋛ Troubleshooting Tips ⋚

If you still struggle with the uncertainty of your worry, try listing all the activities and decisions you make in everyday life that involve an acceptance of uncertainty (e.g., crossing the street and assuming drivers won't run a red light). Practice focusing on whether it is even possible to reduce any further the uncertainty about a future worry. You could also question others about how they think about the uncertainty of their health, relationships, finances, or work. In each case your goal is not eliminating uncertainty (this is impossible) but accepting uncertainty.

CHAPTER SUMMARY

■ Generalized anxiety disorder (GAD) is the second most common anxiety disorder and is characterized by persistent anxiety and excessive, uncontrollable worry about various life concerns.

■ Maladaptive worry involves a narrow focus on exaggerated future threat (catastrophizing), an attempt to reduce uncertainty through futile problem solving and reassurance seeking, and ineffective efforts to stop the worry process.

■ Worry is rarely productive or helpful for chronically anxious people. Instead their unproductive worry involves a preoccupation with imagined, hypothetical, "what if" worst-case scenarios, over which they have minimal control and where failed problem-solving efforts leave them feeling frightened, helpless, and uncertain.

■ Worry is a state of mind, a way of thinking in which distressing intrusive thoughts about threats to valued life goals activate underlying beliefs about future threat and personal helplessness, resulting in a worry process characterized by failed mental control of worry, a search for relief, ineffective problem solving, and "worry about being worried."

■ Defeating unproductive worry begins with discovering your unique worry profile. This involves identifying your main worry concerns, recognizing how you catastrophize the future, determining your core worry beliefs, and specifying maladaptive worry control strategies.

■ The first step in cognitive therapy for worry involves determining whether your worry is about more immediate, realistic concerns. Constructive problem solving is one of the best intervention strategies for reducing the anxiety and worry associated with realistic life problems (e.g., dealing with unemployment, a broken relationship, serious medical illness, loss of a loved one).

■ Most of the worries found in GAD focus on more distant, somewhat abstract, even hypothetical, threatening possibilities in the future (e.g., "whether I'm accepted and loved," "whether I will lose everything and become destitute," "whether I'll die young").

■ Cognitive therapy for worry about more imagined future concerns consists of correcting catastrophic thinking, doing imaginal exposure to the worst possible outcome, repeatedly engaging in structured and direct worry expression, generating a "decatastrophizing plan," correcting maladaptive positive and negative beliefs about worry, reducing worry control efforts, and accepting risk, novelty, and uncertainty.

Resources

Associations

Various professional mental health associations in North America, Europe, and Australia have websites that provide useful information on the latest research and treatment of anxiety for the general public. A few of these sites also provide information on how to locate a competently trained cognitive or cognitive behavior therapist in your region.

United States

Anxiety and Depression Association of America
8701 Georgia Avenue, # 412
Silver Spring, MD 20910
Phone: 240-485-1001
Website: *www.adaa.org*

Association for Behavioral and Cognitive Therapies
305 Seventh Avenue, 16th Floor
New York, NY 10001-6008
Phone: 212-647-1890
Fax: 212-647-1865
Website: *www.abct.org*

Academy of Cognitive Therapy
245 North 15th Street, MS 403
17 New College Building
Department of Psychiatry
Philadelphia, PA 19102
Fax: 215-731-2182
E-mail: *info@academyofct.org*
Website: *www.academyofct.org*

American Psychological Association
750 First Street, NE
Washington, DC 20002-4242
Phone: 800-374-2721
Website: *www.apa.org*

American Psychiatric Association
APA Answer Center
1000 Wilson Boulevard, Suite 1825
Arlington, VA 22209
Phone: 888-35-PSYCH (or 703-907-7300)
E-mail: *apa@psych.org*
Website: *www.psych.org*

Canada

Anxiety Disorders Association of Canada
101-631 Columbia Street
New Westminster, British Columbia
V3M 1A7, Canada
E-mail: *contactus@anxietycanada.ca*
Website: *www.anxietycanada.ca*

Canadian Association of Cognitive and Behavioural Therapies
260 Queen Street West
P.O. Box 60055
Toronto, Ontario
M5V 0C5, Canada
Website: *www.cacbt.ca*

Canadian Psychological Association
141 Laurier Avenue West, Suite 702
Ottawa, Ontario K1P 5J3, Canada
Toll free: 888-472-0657
Fax: 613-237-1674
E-mail: *cpa@cpa.ca*
Website: *www.cpa.ca*

United Kingdom

British Association for Behavioural and Cognitive Psychotherapies
Imperial House, Hornby Street
Bury, Lancaster BL9 5BN, United Kingdom
Phone: +44 0161 705 4304
Fax: +44 0161 705 4306
E-mail: *babcp@babcp.com*
Website: *www.babcp.com*

British Psychological Society
St. Andrews House
48 Princess Road East
Leicester LE1 7DR, United Kingdom
Phone: +44 (0)116 254 9568
Fax: +44 (0)116 227 1314
E-mail: *enquiries@bps.org.uk*
Website: *www.bps.org.uk*

Australia

Australian Association for Cognitive and Behaviour Therapy Ltd.
P.O. Box 4040
Nowra East, NSW 2541, Australia
Fax: +61 07 3041 0415
E-mail: *info@aacbt.org*
Website: *www.aacbt.org*

International

International Association for Cognitive Psychotherapy
www.the-iacp.com

Internet Resources

Anxieties.com
www.anxieties.com

Anxiety Treatment Australia
www.anxietyaustralia.com.au

Anxiety-Panic.com
www.anxiety-panic.com

Anxiety and Depression Association of America
www.adaa.org

Freedom from Fear
www.freedomfromfear.org

International OCD Foundation
www.ocfoundation.org

Internet Mental Health
www.mentalhealth.com

National Alliance on Mental Illness
www.nami.org

National Center for PTSD
www.ptsd.va.gov

National Institute for Health and Care Excellence
www.nice.org.uk

National Institute of Mental Health Anxiety Disorders Publications
www.nimh.nih.gov/health/publications/index.shtml

PTSD Social Support Network
www.ptsd.org

The Panic Center
www.paniccenter.net

Social Anxiety Association
www.socialphobia.org

Social Phobia World
www.socialphobiaworld.com

Recommended Reading

The following are self-help books that offer various types of cognitively related treatments for anxiety and its disorders. These resources vary in their emphasis on cognitive and behavioral strategies for reducing anxiety. Some include alternative strategies for reducing anxiety such as meditation, mindfulness training, and acceptance/commitment approaches. We have also expanded the list to include resources on obsessive–compulsive disorder, posttraumatic stress disorder, and depression.

Anxiety Disorders (General)

Antony, M. M., & Norton, P. J. (2009). *The anti-anxiety workbook*. New York: Guilford Press.

Antony, M. M., & Swinson, R. P. (2008). *When perfect isn't good enough: Strategies for coping with perfectionism* (2nd ed.). Oakland, CA: New Harbinger.

Bourne, E. J. (2003). *Coping with anxiety: 10 simple ways to relieve anxiety, fear, and worry*. Oakland, CA: New Harbinger.

Bourne, E. J. (2005). *The anxiety and phobia workbook* (4th ed.). Oakland, CA: New Harbinger.

Butler, G., & Hope, T. (2007). *Managing your mind: The mental fitness guide*. Oxford, UK: Oxford University Press.

Kennerley, H. (2009). *Overcoming anxiety: A self-help guide using cognitive behavioural techniques*. London: Constable & Robinson.

Kennerley, H. (2006). *Overcoming anxiety self-help course: A 3-part programme based on cognitive behavioural techniques*. London: Constable & Robinson.

Knaus, B. J. (2008). *The cognitive behavioral workbook for anxiety: A step-by-step program*. Oakland, CA: New Harbinger.

Leahy, R. L. (2009). *Anxiety free: Unravel your fears before they unravel you*. Carlsbad, CA: Hays House.

Orsillo, S. M., & Roemer, L. (2011). *The mindful way through anxiety: Break free from chronic worry and reclaim your life*. New York: Guilford Press.

Shafran, R., Egan, S., & Wade, T. (2010). *Overcoming perfectionism: A self-help guide using cognitive behavioural techniques*. London: Constable & Robinson.

Watt, M. C., & Stewart, S. H. (2009). *Overcoming fear of fear: How to reduce anxiety sensitivity*. Oakland, CA: New Harbinger.

Wilding, C., & Milne, A. (2008). *Cognitive behavioural therapy*. London: Hodder Education.

Panic Disorder

Antony, M. M., & McCabe, R. E. (2004). *10 simple solutions to panic: How to overcome panic attacks, calm physical symptoms, and reclaim your life*. Oakland, CA: New Harbinger.

Barlow, D. H., & Craske, M. G. (2007). *Mastery of your anxiety and panic* (4th ed., workbook). New York: Oxford University Press.

Silove, D., & Manicavasagar, V. (2007). *Overcoming panic and agoraphobia self-help course: A 3-part programme based on cognitive behavioural techniques.* London: Constable & Robinson.

Zuercher-White, E. (1997). *An end to panic: Breakthrough techniques for overcoming panic disorder* (2nd ed.). Oakland, CA: New Harbinger.

Social Anxiety Disorder

Antony, M. M. (2004). *10 simple solutions to shyness: How to overcome shyness, social anxiety, and fear of public speaking.* Oakland, CA: New Harbinger.

Antony, M. M., & Swinson, R. P. (2008). *The shyness and social anxiety workbook: Proven, step-by-step techniques for overcoming your fear* (2nd ed.). Oakland, CA: New Harbinger.

Butler, G. (2007). *Overcoming social anxiety and shyness self-help course: A 3-part programme based on cognitive behavioural techniques.* London: Constable & Robinson.

Hope, D. A., Heimberg, R. G., & Turk, C. L. (2006). *Managing social anxiety: A cognitive-behavioral therapy approach.* Oxford: Oxford University Press.

Stein, M. B., & Walker, J. R. (2002) *Triumph over shyness: Conquering shyness and social anxiety.* New York: McGraw-Hill.

Generalized Anxiety Disorder and Worry

Gyoerkoe, K. L., & Wiegartz, P. S. (2006). *10 simple solutions to worry: How to calm your mind, relax your body, and reclaim your life.* Oakland, CA: New Harbinger.

Hazlett-Stevens, H. (2005). *Women who worry too much: How to stop worry and anxiety from ruining relationships, work, and fun.* Oakland, CA: New Harbinger.

Leahy, R. L. (2005). *The worry cure: Seven steps to stop worry from stopping you.* New York: Harmony Books.

Meares, K., & Freeston, M. (2008). *Overcoming worry: A self-help guide using cognitive behavioural techniques.* London: Constable & Robinson.

Rygh, J. L., & Sanderson, W. C. (2004). *Treating generalized anxiety disorder: Evidence-based strategies, tools, and techniques.* New York: Guilford Press.

Obsessive–Compulsive Disorder

Abramowitz, J. S. (2009). *Getting over OCD: A 10-step workbook for taking back your life.* New York: Guilford Press.

Purdon, C. L. & Clark, D. A. (2005). *Overcoming obsessive thoughts: How to gain control of your OCD.* Oakland, CA: New Harbinger.

Steketee, G. (1999). *Overcoming obsessive–compulsive disorder: A behavioral and cognitive protocol for treatment of OCD.* Oakland, CA: New Harbinger.

Steketee, G., & Frost, R. O. (2007). *Compulsive hoarding and acquiring workbook.* Oxford, UK: Oxford University Press.

Veale, D., & Willson, R. (2005). *Overcoming obsessive compulsive disorder: A self-help guide using cognitive behavioural techniques.* London: Constable & Robinson.

Posttraumatic Stress Disorders

Najavits, L. M. (2002). *Seeking safety: A treatment manual for PTSD and substance abuse.* New York: Guilford Press.

Scott, M. J. (2008). *Moving on after trauma: A guide for survivors, family and friends.* London: Routledge.

Zayfert, C., & DeViva, J. C. (2011). *When someone you love suffers from posttraumatic stress: What to expect and what you can do.* New York: Guilford Press.

Depression

Addis, M. E., & Martell, C. R. (2004). *Overcoming depression one step at a time: The new behavioral activation approach to getting your life back.* Oakland, CA: New Harbinger.

Bieling, P. J., & Antony, M. M. (2003). *Ending the depression cycle.* Oakland, CA: New Harbinger.

Fennell, M. (2011). *Boost your confidence: Improving self-esteem step-by-step.* London: Constable & Robinson.

Greenberger, D., & Padesky, C. A. (1995). *Mind over mood: Change how you feel by changing the way you think.* New York: Guilford Press.

Leahy, R. L. (2010). *Beat the blues before they beat you: How to overcome depression.* Carlsbad, CA: Hays House.

Williams, M., Teasdale, J., Segal, Z., & Kabat-Zinn, J. (2007). *The mindful way through depression: Freeing yourself from chronic unhappiness.* New York: Guilford Press.

References

1. The calculation for anxiety disorders is based on a lifetime prevalence rate of 28.8% reported in Kessler, R. C., Berglund, P., Demler, O., Robertson, M. S., & Walters, E. E. (2005). Lifetime prevalence and age-of-onset distributions of *DSM-IV* disorders in the National Comorbidity Survey Replication. *Archives of General Psychiatry, 62,* 593–602.

2. National Institute of Anxiety and Stress, Inc (2009). *Famous people with anxiety.* Retrieved August 6, 2009 from *www.conqueranxiety.com/famous-people-with-anxiety. asp.*

3. Beck, A. T. (1967). *Depression: Causes and treatment.* Philadelphia: University of Pennsylvania Press.

4. Beck, A. T., & Emery, G. (with Greenberg, R. L.). (1985). *Anxiety disorders and phobias: A cognitive perspective.* New York: Basic Books.

5. Clark, D. A., & Beck, A. T. (2010). *Cognitive therapy of anxiety disorders: Science and practice.* New York: Guilford Press.

6. Butler, A. C., Chapman, J. F., Forman, E. M., & Beck, A. T. (2006). The empirical status of cognitive-behavioral therapy: A review of meta-analyses. *Clinical Psychology Review, 26,* 17–31.

7. Epp, A. M., Dobson, K. S. & Cottraux, J. (2009). Applications of individual cognitive-behavioral therapy to specific disorders. In G. O. Gabbard (Ed.), *Textbook of psychotherapeutic treatments* (pp. 239–262). Washington, DC: American Psychiatric Publishing.

8. Hollon, S. D., Stewart, M. O., & Strunk, D. (2006). Enduring effects for cognitive behavior therapy in the treatment of depression and anxiety. *Annual Review of Psychology, 57,* 285–315.

9. American Psychiatric Association. (1998). Practice guidelines for the treatment of patients with panic disorder. *American Journal of Psychiatry, 155*(Suppl.), 1–34.

10. Chambless, D. L., Baker, M. J., Baucom, D. H., Beutler, L. E., Calhoun, K. S., Crits-

Christoph, P., et al. (1998). Update on empirically validated therapies II. *The Clinical Psychologist, 51,* 3–16.

11. McIntosh, A., Cohen, A., Turnbull, N., Esmonde, L., Dennis, P., Eatock, J., et al. (2004). *Clinical guidelines and evidence review for panic disorder and generalised anxiety disorder.* Sheffield, UK: University of Sheffield/London: National Collaborating Centre for Primary Care.

12. Beck, J. S. (1995). *Cognitive therapy: Basics and beyond.* New York: Guilford Press.

13. Beck, A. T., Rush, A. J., Shaw, B. F., & Emery, G. (1979). *Cognitive therapy of depression.* New York: Guilford Press.

14. American Psychiatric Association. (2000). *Diagnostic and statistical manual of mental disorders* (4th ed., text rev.). Washington, DC: Author.

15. Antony, M. M., & Norton, P. J. (2009). *The anti-anxiety workbook: Proven strategies to overcome worry, phobias, panic, and obsessions.* New York: Guilford Press.

16. Mathews, A., & MacLeod, C. (2005). Cognitive vulnerability to emotional disorders. *Annual Review of Clinical Psychology, 1,* 167–195.

17. MacLeod, C. (1999). Anxiety and anxiety disorders. In T. Dalgleish & M. Power (Eds.), *Handbook of cognition and emotion* (pp. 447–477). Chichester, UK: Wiley.

18. Craske, M. G., & Barlow, D. H. (2006). *Mastery of your anxiety and worry: Workbook* (2nd ed.). Oxford, UK: Oxford University Press.

19. Reiss, S., & McNally, R. J. (1985). Expectancy model of fear. In S. Reiss & R. R. Bootzin (Eds.), *Theoretical issues in behavior therapy* (pp. 107–121). Orlando, FL: Academic Press.

20. Taylor, S. (1995). Anxiety sensitivity: Theoretical perspectives and recent findings. *Behaviour Research and Therapy, 33,* 243–258.

21. Dugas, M. J., Buhr, K., & Ladouceur, R. (2004). The role of intolerance of uncertainty in etiology and maintenance. In R. G. Heimberg, C. L. Turk, & D. S. Mennin (Eds.), *Generalized anxiety disorder: Advances in research and practice* (pp. 143–163). New York: Guilford Press.

22. Salkovskis, P. M. (1996). Avoidance behavior is motivated by threat belief: A possible resolution of the cognitive-behavior debate. In P. M. Salkovskis (Ed.), *Trends in cognitive and behavioral therapies* (pp. 25–41). Chichester, UK: Wiley.

23. Lohr, J. M., Olatunji, B. O., & Sawchuk, C. N. (2007). A functional analysis of danger and safety signals in anxiety disorders. *Clinical Psychology Review, 27,* 114–126.

24. Mental fitness: What is it? Retrieved November 18, 2009, *www.riley.army.mil/documents/DaggersEdge/091030144723.pdf.*

25. Kazantzis, N., Whittington, C., & Dattilio, F. (2010). Meta-analysis of homework effects

in cognitive and behavioral therapy: A replication and extension. *Clinical Psychology: Science and Practice, 17,* 144–156.

26. Lambert, M. J., Harmon, S. C., & Slade, K. (2007). Directions for research on homework. In N. Kazantzis & L. L'Abate (Eds.), *Handbook of homework assignments in psychotherapy: Research, practice, and prevention* (pp. 407–423). New York: Springer.

27. Gray, J. A. (1971). *The psychology of fear and success.* London: Weidenfeld and Nicolson.

28. Leahy, R. L. (2009). *Anxiety free: Unravel your fears before they unravel you.* Carlsbad, CA: Hay House.

29. Merriam-Webster's Online Dictionary. Retrieved January 23, 2010, *www.merriam-webster.com/dictionary.*

30. Abramowitz, J. S., Deacon, B. J., & Whiteside, S. P. H. (2011). *Exposure therapy for anxiety: Principles and practice.* New York: Guilford Press.

31. Barlow, D. H. (2002). *Anxiety and its disorders: The nature and treatment of anxiety and panic* (2nd ed.). New York: Guilford Press.

32. Clark, D. M. (1986). A cognitive approach to panic. *Behaviour Research and Therapy, 24,* 461–470.

33. Norton, G. R., Dorward, J., & Cox, B. J. (1986). Factors associated with panic attacks in nonclinical subjects. *Behavior Therapy, 17,* 239–252.

34. Brown, T. A., & Deagle, E. A. (1992). Structured interview assessment of nonclinical panic. *Behavior Therapy, 23,* 75–85.

35. Reiss, S., Peterson, R. A., Gursky, D. M., & McNally, R. J. (1986). Anxiety sensitivity, anxiety frequency and the prediction of fearfulness. *Behaviour Research and Therapy, 24,* 1–8.

36. Taylor, S. (1995). Anxiety sensitivity: Theoretical perspectives and recent findings. *Behaviour Research and Therapy, 33,* 243–258.

37. McNally, R. J. (2002). Anxiety sensitivity and panic disorder. *Biological Psychiatry, 52,* 938–946.

38. Taylor, S., Zvolensky, M. J., Cox, B. J., Deacon, B., Heimberg, R. G., Ledley, D. R., et al. (2007). Robust dimensions of anxiety sensitivity: Development and initial validation of the Anxiety Sensitivity Index–3. *Psychological Assessment, 19,* 176–188.

39. National Institute of Mental Health. (2008). *The numbers count: Mental disorders in America.* Retrieved April 23, 2010, from *www.nimh.nih.gov/health/publications/the-numbers-count-mental-disorders-in-america.*

40. Henderson, L., & Zimbardo, P. (1999). Shyness. In H. S. Friedman (Ed.), *Encyclopedia of mental health* (Vol 3, pp. 497–509), San Diego, CA: Academic Press.

41. Fehm, L., Beesdo, K., Jacobi, F., & Fiedler, A. (2008). Social anxiety disorder above and below the diagnostic threshold: Prevalence, comorbidity and impairment in the general population. *Social Psychiatry and Psychiatric Epidemiology, 43,* 257–265.

42. Clark, D. M. (2001). A cognitive perspective on social phobia. In W. R. Crozier and L. E. Alden (Eds.), *International handbook of social anxiety: Concepts, research, and interventions relating to the self and shyness* (pp. 405–430). New York: Wiley.

43. Fisher, P. L. (2006). The efficacy of psychological treatments for generalized anxiety disorder. In G. C. L. Davey & A. Wells (Eds.), *Worry and its psychological disorders: Theory, assessment and treatment* (pp. 359–377). Chichester, UK: Wiley.

44. Craske, M. G., & Barlow, D. H. (2006). *Mastery of your anxiety and worry: Workbook* (2nd ed.). Oxford, UK: Oxford University Press.

45. Dugas, M. J., Ladouceur, R., Léger, E., Freeston, M. H., Langlois F., Provencher, M. D., et al. (2003). Group cognitive-behavioral therapy for generalized anxiety disorders: Treatment outcome and long-term follow-up. *Journal of Consulting and Clinical Psychology, 71,* 821–825.

46. Gosselin, P., Ladouceur, R., Morin, C. M., Dugas, M. J., & Baillargeon, L. (2006). Benzodiazepine discontinuation among adults with GAD: A randomized trial of cognitive-behavioral therapy. *Journal of Consulting and Clinical Psychology, 74,* 908–919.

47. Wegner, D. M. (1994). The ironic processes of mental control. *Psychological Review, 101,* 34–52.

48. Leahy, R. L. (2005). *The worry cure: Seven steps to stop worry from stopping you.* New York: Harmony Books.

49. Wells, A. (2009). *Metacognitive therapy for anxiety and depression.* New York: Guilford Press.

50. Borkovec, T. D., Alcaine, O. M., & Behar, E. (2004). Avoidance theory of worry and generalized anxiety disorder. In R. G. Heimberg, C. L. Turk, & D. S. Mennin (Eds.), *Generalized anxiety disorder: Advances in research and practice* (pp. 77–108). New York: Guilford Press.

51. Koerner, N., & Dugas, M. J. (2006). A cognitive model of generalized anxiety disorder: The role of intolerance of uncertainty. In G. C. L. Davey & A. Wells (Eds.), *Worry and its psychological disorders: Theory, assessment and treatment* (pp. 202–216). Chichester, UK: Wiley.

52. Robichaud, M., & Dugas, M. J. (2006). A cognitive-behavioral treatment targeting intolerance of uncertainty. In G. C. L. Davey & A. Wells (Eds.), *Worry and its psychological disorders: Theory, assessment and treatment* (pp. 289–304). Chichester, UK: Wiley.

Index

About the Authors

David A. Clark, PhD, is Professor of Psychology at the University of New Brunswick, Canada, where he also has had a private practice for 25 years. Dr. Clark is a widely recognized authority on cognitive behavior therapy for anxiety and depression and is the author of numerous books, including *The Mood Repair ToolKit*. He is a Fellow of the Canadian Psychological Association and Founding Fellow of the Academy of Cognitive Therapy.

Aaron T. Beck, MD, is University Professor Emeritus of Psychiatry at the University of Pennsylvania School of Medicine and President of the Beck Institute for Cognitive Behavior Therapy. A world-renowned researcher, educator, and practicing psychiatrist, Dr. Beck is the founder of cognitive therapy. He has been honored with numerous awards, including the Lasker Award for Clinical Medical Research and research awards from both the American Psychiatric Association and the American Psychological Association.

Together, Drs. Clark and Beck are the authors of a related professional book, *Cognitive Therapy of Anxiety Disorders*, also published by Guilford.